HIGH-PROTEIN

PANCAKES

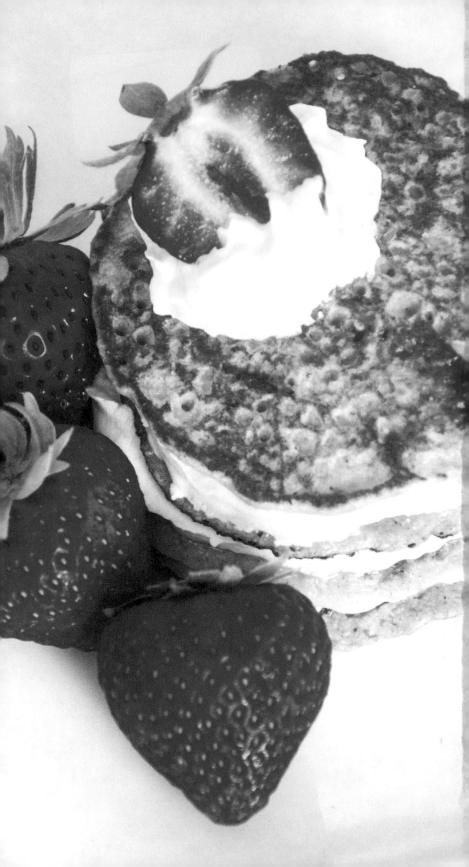

PAMELA BRAUN

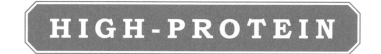

HIGH-PROTEIN

PANCAKES

STRENGTH-BUILDING RECIPES
FOR EVERYDAY HEALTH

THE COUNTRYMAN PRESS

A division of W. W. Norton & Company

Independent Publishers Since 1923

For information about permission to reproduce selections from this
book, write to Permissions, The Countryman Press,
500 Fifth Avenue, New York, NY 10110

For information about special discounts for bulk purchases,
please contact W. W. Norton Special Sales at
specialsales@wwnorton.com or 800-233-4830

Manufacturing by Versa Press
Book design by Chin-Yee Lai
Production manager: Devon Zahn

Library of Congress Cataloging-in-Publication Data
Names: Braun, Pamela, author.
Title: High-protein pancakes : strength-building
recipes for everyday health / Pamela Braun.
Description: New York, NY : Countryman Press,
a division of W. W. Norton & Company, Independent
Publishers Since 1923, [2017] | Includes index.
Identifiers: LCCN 2016047988 | ISBN 9781682680230 (pbk.)
Subjects: LCSH: Pancakes, waffles, etc. |
High-protein diet—Recipes | LCGFT: Cookbooks.
Classification: LCC TX770.P34 B73 2017 | DDC 641.81/53—dc23
LC record available at https://lccn.loc.gov/2016047988

The Countryman Press
www.countrymanpress.com

A division of W. W. Norton & Company, Inc.
500 Fifth Avenue, New York, NY 10110
www.wwnorton.com

10 9 8 7 6 5 4 3 2 1

CONTENTS

INTRODUCTION

Pancakes. Is there any other food so synonymous with breakfast? Is there one more universally liked than pancakes? I would argue the answer to both of these questions is no. The pancake is the king of breakfast.

The biggest downside to eating pancakes—aside from when the stack is gone—is that they can be carbohydrate lumps that sit like rocks in your stomach. Often heavy and dense, they may make you want to go back to bed once you've finished eating them. That's fine if it's going to be a lazy weekend, but what if you've got things to do? You probably grab a bowl of cereal or some scrambled eggs instead. But what if I were to tell you that on those run-around kind of days you could have your (pan)cake and eat it too? These pancake recipes were developed with busy lives in mind. They're loaded with protein so you don't get that carb-loaded, bloated, sleepy feeling, and you can keep going through your day.

These pancake recipes were created with flours and other ingredients that are naturally higher in protein than what pancakes are usually made from. I did not use protein powder in them. If you would really like to boost the protein in these recipes, you could add a scoop of your favorite protein powder for even more protein in each serving.

Some of the recipes in this book make four servings of pancakes. If you aren't feeding that many people, no worries—you can freeze the pancakes for later. Just make the pancakes as you normally would. Let them cool completely, then layer them between pieces of waxed paper. Slide the pancakes into a zip-top bag and place them in the freezer. To re-heat, you can do a couple of things. You can let them thaw, then heat them in a skillet or you can pop the frozen pancakes into the microwave for a minute. Just remember to remove the waxed paper regardless of which method you use. If there is a topping that goes with the recipe of pancakes you are freezing, you can make up the topping and refrigerate it for up to a week. Otherwise, you'll need to make the topping fresh when you're re-heating the pancakes.

INGREDIENTS

The ingredients in some of these pancakes may sound strange (they aren't your typical all-purpose flour, egg, and milk recipes), but they give the pancakes a boost of protein.

Like I said, I didn't use protein powder in any of these pancake recipes. Ingredients like spelt flour, oatmeal, kefir, and cottage cheese provide a serious serving of protein and are a lot less processed. It isn't that I don't like protein powder—I just wanted to use whole ingredients to deliver the protein in these pancakes.

These ingredients are readily available either in your local grocery store (and if they don't carry something, ask them to order it) or online. It was important to me to create recipes that could be easily duplicated in your kitchen.

TIPS FOR THE PERFECT PANCAKE

Fresh ingredients are the best ingredients. It makes a big difference in the finished pancake if your flour, baking soda, baking powder, eggs, and milk/nut milk are fresh. Especially the baking soda and baking powder. Old products can leave you with flat, crepe-like discs instead of fluffy pancakes.

For the fruit pancakes, it is best to use fresh, in-season produce. If that's not possible, you can use frozen, thawed fruit. I like to use fresh fruit because the flavor is a bit better, especially when it comes to peaches.

Don't overmix the batter. Mix the dry ingredients together in one bowl in order to thoroughly mix the leavening agent(s) throughout the mix. Then add the wet ingredients and mix those in until everything is wet. It's okay if your batter is a little lumpy. If you overmix the batter, you'll develop the gluten and your pancakes will be tough.

Some of these recipes call for using a blender to mix the ingredients. I used a high-speed blender, but you can use any blender that you have. You only need to blend the ingredients until they're broken down and thoroughly mixed. This doesn't take long.

While I know it can be really convenient to make your pancake batter in advance, the ingredients in these pancakes don't work as well when you make them ahead of time.

The batter has a tendency to absorb all of the moisture and become too thick to pour. I recommend you make the batter when you're ready to make and eat the pancakes.

I used a griddle to prepare my pancakes, but you can use a frying pan if that's what you have. If you use a frying pan, you may not be able to make as many at the same time so it will just take you a bit longer to cook all the pancakes.

You'll notice that the recipes call for spray oil. This is vegetable oil. I don't use the traditional butter to make my pancakes because butter has a low smoke point and can cause your pancakes to burn before they're cooked through. The vegetable oil has a higher smoke point, so your pancakes are able to cook through and not burn as easily. Some of these pancakes have a really wet batter and take a little extra time to cook (it's noted in the recipe) so the vegetable oil is perfect in this case. You will need to re-spray the pan or griddle in between each batch of pancakes so that they don't stick.

I also used a ¼ cup when measuring out and pouring my batter. The number of pancakes listed with each recipe is based on a full ¼-cup measure, although you may get more pancakes if you don't fill your measuring cup as full. Make sure that all of your pancakes are uniform in size. This way they will all cook at the same rate.

You'll know when it's time to flip the pancakes by watching the bubbles that form as well as the edges of the pancakes. The bubbles form deep holes and the edges begin to look dry when the pancakes are ready to be flipped. This does take a little practice, so don't be discouraged if your first few pancakes come out over- or undercooked.

Pancakes taste their best when they are hot. As you take them off the griddle or pan, place them onto an oven-safe plate, then place the plate into an oven preheated to 275°F. This will keep them nice and warm for serving.

Creating the recipes for this book has been a delicious adventure. I hope you enjoy eating these pancakes as much as I enjoyed making them.

All nutritional information is per serving and is approximate.

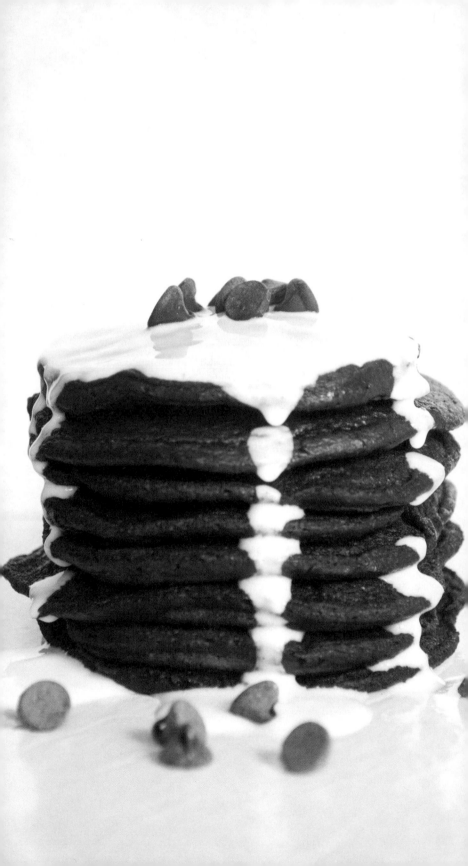

RED VELVET PANCAKES

Topping

½ cup plain kefir

2 tablespoons powdered sugar

Pancakes

1¾ cups old-fashioned rolled oats

3 tablespoons cocoa powder (unsweetened)

1½ teaspoons baking powder

1 teaspoon baking soda

¼ teaspoon salt

3 tablespoons maple syrup

2 tablespoons coconut oil (melted)

1½ cups 2% low-fat milk

1 large egg

1 teaspoon red food coloring

Chocolate shavings or chips, for serving

These Red Velvet Pancakes aren't as rich as their namesake cake but have the same flavor and a lot more protein. They're rich and chocolatey and the topping tastes a lot like cream cheese frosting. Top them off with chocolate shavings or chips for even more chocolate flavor.

1. For the topping, add both ingredients to a small bowl and stir until combined. Set aside.
2. For the pancakes, add all items to a high-speed blender and blitz on high to liquefy. Make sure everything is well blended.
3. Let the batter rest for 5 to 10 minutes. This allows all of the ingredients to come together and gives the batter a better consistency.
4. Spray a non-stick skillet or griddle generously with vegetable oil and heat over medium heat.
5. Once the skillet is hot, add the batter using a ¼-cup measuring cup and pour the batter into the skillet to make the pancake. Use the measuring cup to help shape the pancake.
6. Cook until the sides appear set and bubbles form in the middle (about 2 to 3 minutes), then flip the pancake.
7. Once the pancake is cooked on that side, remove pancake from the heat and place on a plate.
8. Continue these steps with the rest of the batter.
9. Stack and serve with topping and chocolate chips.

Protein 12 grams | Carbs 43 grams | Calories 318

DARK CHOCOLATE PANCAKES

Filling

1 cup dark chocolate chips (at least 60% cocoa)

½ cup heavy whipping cream

Pancakes

1¾ cups old-fashioned rolled oats

1½ teaspoons baking powder

1 teaspoon baking soda

½ teaspoon cinnamon

¼ teaspoon salt

2 tablespoons coconut oil (melted)

1 tablespoon maple syrup

1 teaspoon vanilla extract

1½ cups 2% low-fat milk

1 large egg

Powdered sugar and sliced strawberries, for serving

Dark chocolate pancakes are your excuse for eating dessert first—I mean first thing in the morning. They're so rich and full of chocolate you won't believe you get to have these for breakfast. They take a little extra prep work but the end result is well worth the time you spend on them. And yes, the strawberries are practically mandatory with these pancakes . . . they just taste so good together.

For the Filling

1. Pour the chocolate chips into a bowl and pour the cream into a small saucepan.
2. Heat the cream until the edges bubble, then pour over the chocolate.
3. Let the chocolate sit for 2 minutes (this helps the chocolate melt), then stir to form a thick ganache.
4. Line a baking sheet with parchment paper.
5. Oil the inside of a 2-inch round cookie cutter.
6. Pour 1 teaspoon of the chocolate into the cookie cutter and spread it out so that it forms a circle. Remove the cutter and continue making ganache circles (should yield about six).
7. Place the baking sheet into the freezer and freeze the ganache for at least 4 hours to overnight.

For the Pancakes

1. Add all items, except the strawberries, to a high-speed blender and blitz on high to liquefy. Make sure everything is well blended.
2. Pour the batter into a bowl and let it rest for 2 to 3 minutes. This allows the batter to thicken up so that it can hold the chocolate when you flip the pancakes.

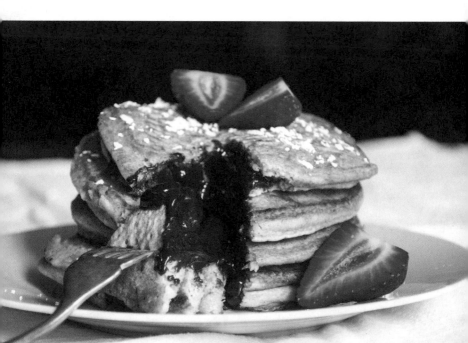

3. Spray a non-stick skillet or griddle generously with vegetable oil and heat over medium heat.
4. Once the skillet is hot, use a ¼-cup measuring cup to pour the batter into a skillet.
5. Gently spread the batter into a round shape with the measuring cup.
6. Place 1 frozen ganache circle (flipped so that the lumpy side is down) in the center of the batter and gently press it into the batter. Pour more batter over ganache circle just until it is covered.
7. Cook until the batter is dry to the touch (about 3 to 4 minutes), then carefully flip the pancake.
8. Continue cooking until the other side of the pancake is golden brown.
9. Once the pancake is cooked on that side, remove the pancake from the heat and place on a plate.
10. Continue with remaining batter and chocolate.
11. Serve pancakes with powdered sugar and sliced strawberries.

Protein 20 grams | Carbs 98 grams | Calories 1,024

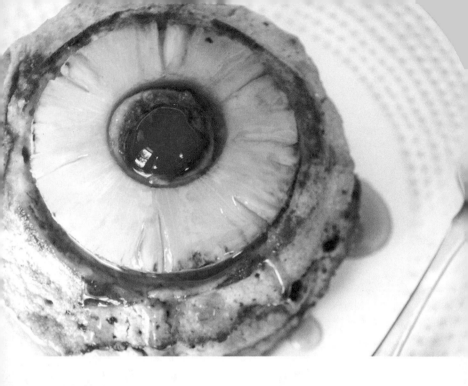

PINEAPPLE UPSIDE-DOWN PANCAKES

1 (20-ounce) can pineapple rings (drained)
1¾ cups old-fashioned rolled oats
1½ teaspoons baking powder
1 teaspoon baking soda
½ teaspoon cinnamon
¼ teaspoon salt
2 tablespoons maple syrup

2 tablespoons coconut oil (melted)
1½ cups 2% low-fat milk
1 large egg
Brown sugar
Maraschino cherries (de-stemmed and cut in half), for serving

1. Place the pineapple rings on a double layer of paper towels to drain excess liquid.
2. Add all items, except pineapple, brown sugar, and maraschino cherries, to a high-speed blender and blitz on high to liquefy. Make sure everything is well blended.
3. Pour batter into a bowl and let it rest for 2 to 3 minutes. This allows the batter to thicken up so that it can hold those pineapple rings when you flip the pancakes.
4. Spray a non-stick skillet or griddle generously with vegetable oil and heat over medium heat.
5. Once the skillet is hot, use a ¼-cup measuring cup to pour the batter into the pan. Gently spread batter into a round shape with the measuring cup.
6. Place pineapple ring in the center of the batter and gently press it into the batter. Lightly sprinkle some brown sugar directly onto the pineapple ring.
7. Cook until the batter is dry to the touch (about 3 to 4 minutes), then carefully flip the pancake.
8. Continue cooking until the pineapple is good and caramelized.
9. Once the pancake is cooked on that side, remove the pancake from the heat and place on a plate.
10. Continue with remaining batter and pineapple rings.
11. Serve each pancake with a maraschino cherry placed in the center of the pineapple.

Protein 9 grams | Carbs 46 grams | Calories 327

These Pineapple Upside-Down Pancakes taste just like pineapple upside-down cake. They've got that great tropical pineapple flavor mixed with caramelized brown sugar and they're even topped with maraschino cherries. Add maple syrup for a bit more sweetness.

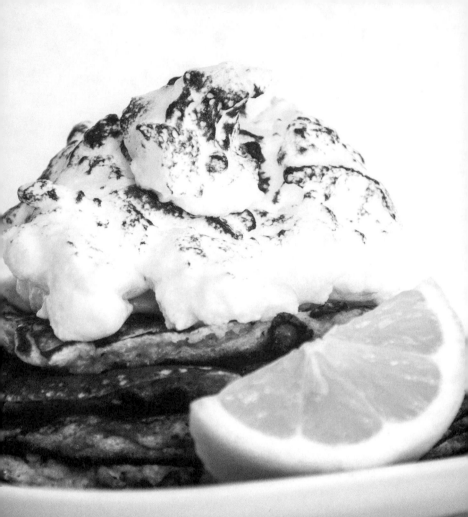

Lemon Meringue Pancakes. Yes, you read that right: Lemon Meringue Pancakes. These pancakes have a subtle lemon flavor, so when you top them with the meringue it makes for a light and fluffy bite of deliciousness. If you want to amp up the lemon flavor, just top the stack with lemon zest.

LEMON MERINGUE PANCAKES

Meringue

4 large egg whites

3 tablespoons sugar

Pancakes

2 eggs

½ cup cottage cheese

½ teaspoon vanilla extract

1 tablespoon honey

¼ cup spelt flour

½ teaspoon baking powder

¼ teaspoon baking soda

2 teaspoons sugar-free lemon Jell-O mix

For the Meringue

1. Add the egg whites to a mixing bowl and beat until soft peaks form. Soft peaks happen when you pull the beaters from the mixture and the peak forms but falls over quickly.
2. Add the sugar to the egg whites and continue to beat until stiff peaks form. Stiff peaks happen when you pull the beaters from the mixture and the peak forms and holds its shape.
3. Set the meringue aside.

For the Pancakes

1. Whisk the eggs, cottage cheese, vanilla, and honey together and set aside.
2. In another bowl, whisk the dry ingredients together until well combined.

Continued

3. Add the wet ingredients to the dry ingredients and whisk until thoroughly combined.
4. Spray a non-stick skillet or griddle generously with vegetable oil and heat over medium heat.
5. Once the skillet is hot, add the batter using a ¼-cup measuring cup and pour the batter into the skillet to make the pancake. Use the measuring cup to help shape the pancake.
6. Cook until the sides appear set and bubbles form in the middle (about 2 to 3 minutes), then flip the pancake.
7. Once the pancake is cooked on that side, remove pancake from the heat and place on a plate.
8. Continue these steps with the rest of the batter.
9. Top pancakes with the meringue.
10. To toast the meringue you can either use a torch to lightly brown the edges or you can pop the topped pancakes under a hot broiler for 2 to 3 minutes.

Protein 23 grams | Carbs 22 grams | Calories 289

CINNAMON ROLL PANCAKES

MAKES 8 PANCAKES | SERVES 4

Cashew Cream Cheese Topping

1 cup raw cashews
⅓ cup water
2 tablespoons honey
1 teaspoon apple cider vinegar

1 teaspoon lemon juice
½ teaspoon vanilla extract
½ teaspoon kosher salt

Cinnamon Filling

½ cup brown sugar
4 tablespoons butter, melted

3 teaspoons cinnamon

Pancakes

1¾ cups old-fashioned rolled
  oats
1½ teaspoons baking powder
1 teaspoon baking soda
½ teaspoon cinnamon
¼ teaspoon salt

2 tablespoons coconut oil,
  melted
1 tablespoon maple syrup
1 large egg
1 teaspoon vanilla extract
1½ cups 2% low-fat milk

For the Cashew Cream Cheese Topping

1. Soak cashews in water overnight.
2. Drain cashews, then add them to a blender along with the rest of the ingredients.
3. Blitz the cashew mixture until it's creamy and has no lumps.
4. Scrape the topping into a small-lidded container and set it aside.

Continued

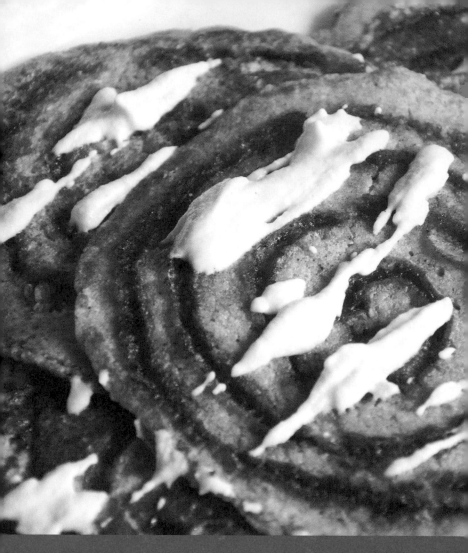

If you like cinnamon rolls, you won't be able to stop eating these Cinnamon Roll Pancakes. It's as if you sliced up a cinnamon roll and toasted it on the stovetop. Topped with a lightly sweet glaze made from cashews, one bite and you'll be in cinnamon heaven.

For the Cinnamon Filling

1. Add all of the ingredients together and stir to combine, making sure that you have broken down any lumps.
2. Pour this mixture into a sandwich bag. You're going to cut the corner tip off the bag and use it as a squeeze bag to pipe the cinnamon swirl onto the pancakes.

For the Pancakes

1. Add all of the ingredients to a blender. The melted coconut oil might harden up when combined with colder ingredients, so you can slightly warm the milk to help prevent this from happening if you'd like.
2. Blitz everything in the blender until you have a smooth liquid.
3. Pour pancake mixture into a large bowl.
4. Let batter rest for 5 to 10 minutes. This allows all of the ingredients to come together and gives the batter a better consistency.
5. Spray a non-stick skillet or griddle generously with vegetable oil and heat over medium heat.
6. Once the skillet is hot, add batter using a ¼-cup measuring cup and pour the batter onto the skillet to make the pancake. Gently spread the batter into a round shape with the measuring cup.
7. Cut the tip from the bag of Cinnamon Filling and squeeze a cinnamon swirl onto the pancake.
8. Cook until the sides appear set and bubbles form in the middle (about 2 to 3 minutes), then flip the pancake.
9. Once the pancake is cooked on that side, remove pancake from the heat and place on a plate.
10. Continue these steps with the rest of the batter.
11. Serve pancakes with the Cashew Cream Cheese Topping.

Protein 19 grams | Carbs 59 grams | Calories 713

KEFIR PANCAKES

1½ cups spelt flour
1½ teaspoons baking powder
1 teaspoon baking soda
½ teaspoon salt
2 tablespoons coconut oil,
    melted

2 large eggs, beaten
¼ cup 2% low-fat milk
1¼ cups plain kefir, slightly
    warmed
¼ cup maple syrup
Blueberries, for serving (optional)

1. Add the flour, baking powder, baking soda, and salt in a large bowl and whisk to thoroughly combine.
2. Add the remaining ingredients to another bowl and whisk to thoroughly combine. The melted coconut oil might harden up when combined with colder ingredients, so you can slightly warm the milk to help prevent this from happening if you'd like.
3. Pour the wet ingredients into the dry ingredients and whisk to combine until all the ingredients are wet.

Kefir has become popular in the health food arena for its probiotic properties as well as a wealth of vitamins and nutrients. While it's a liquid made from milk, it tastes more like yogurt than plain ol' milk. Kefir also contains a good amount of protein in each serving. These hearty pancakes take advantage of that protein and have just a hint of kefir tang in each delicious bite. Top them with fruit and maple syrup for a great start to your day.

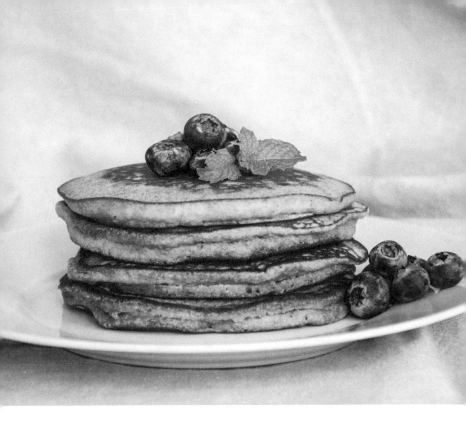

4. Let the batter rest for 2 to 3 minutes. This allows all of the ingredients to come together and gives the batter a better consistency.
5. Spray a non-stick skillet or griddle generously with vegetable oil and heat over medium heat.
6. Once the skillet is hot, add the batter using a ¼-cup measuring cup and pour the batter into the skillet to make the pancake. Use the measuring cup to help shape the pancake.
7. Cook until the sides appear set and bubbles form in the middle (about 2 to 3 minutes), then flip the pancake.
8. Once the pancake is cooked on that side, remove pancake from the heat and place on a plate.
9. Continue these steps with the rest of the batter. Serve with blueberries, if desired.

Protein 13 grams | Carbs 38 grams | Calories 319 grams

KEFIR PANCAKES

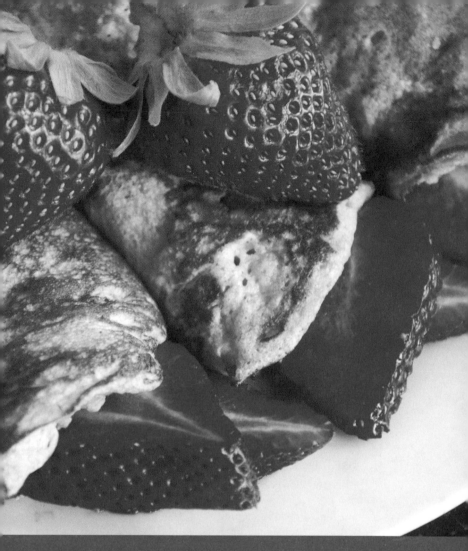

Back in the day, cottage cheese was pretty much reserved for the "dieter's plate" at a restaurant. Cottage cheese might not be an item on your regular menu, but after you have these pancakes I'm betting it will be. The pancakes are light and fluffy and have a great flavor from the cottage cheese.

COTTAGE CHEESE PANCAKES

¼ cup spelt flour
½ teaspoon baking powder
¼ teaspoon baking soda
⅛ teaspoon cinnamon
⅛ teaspoon salt

2 large eggs, beaten
½ cup 2% low-fat cottage cheese
1 tablespoon honey
½ teaspoon vanilla extract
Strawberries, for serving (optional)

1. Add all of the dry ingredients to a bowl and whisk until well combined.
2. In a separate bowl, whisk the wet ingredients together.
3. Add wet ingredients to the dry ingredients and whisk to thoroughly combine them.
4. Let the batter rest for 5 to 10 minutes. This allows all of the ingredients to come together and gives you a better consistency for the batter.
5. Spray a non-stick skillet or griddle generously with vegetable oil and heat over medium heat.
6. Once the skillet is hot, add the batter using a ¼-cup measuring cup and pour the batter into the skillet to make the pancake. Use the measuring cup to help shape the pancake.
7. Cook until the sides appear set and bubbles form in the middle (about 2 to 3 minutes), then flip the pancake.
8. Once the pancake is cooked on that side, remove pancake from the heat and place on a plate.
9. Continue these steps with the rest of the batter. Serve with strawberries, if desired.

Note:
This batter is a little bit runnier than your typical batter, so you might need to use a fork in addition to the spatula to assist in flipping them.

Protein 15 grams | Carbs 22 grams | Calories 211

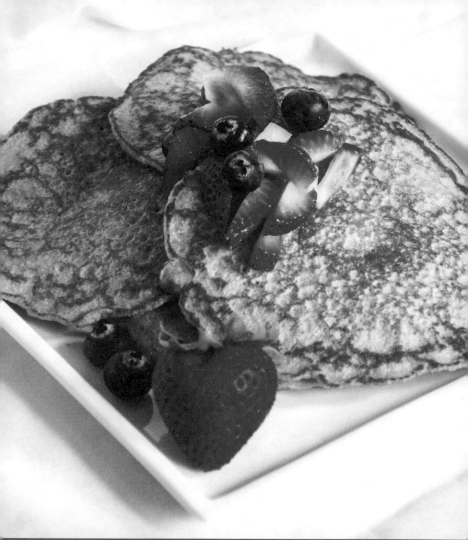

Oatmeal . . . it's what's for breakfast. Except now it's not something to eat out of a bowl— it's something to top with butter and maple syrup. Oatmeal has a surprising amount of protein in it and it's the backbone for these delicious pancakes. There's a touch of sweetness from the maple syrup in these, so you can just top them off with fruit if you don't want to go the butter-and-syrup route.

HIGH-PROTEIN PANCAKES

OATMEAL PANCAKES

1¾ cups old-fashioned rolled oats
1½ teaspoons baking powder
1 teaspoon baking soda
½ teaspoon cinnamon
¼ teaspoon salt
2 tablespoons coconut oil, melted

1 tablespoon maple syrup
1 large egg
1 teaspoon vanilla extract
1½ cups 2% low-fat milk
Strawberries and blueberries, for serving (optional)

1. Add all of the ingredients to a blender. The melted coconut oil might harden up when combined with colder ingredients, so you can slightly warm the milk to help prevent this from happening if you'd like.
2. Blitz everything in the blender until you have a smooth liquid.
3. Pour the pancake mixture into a large bowl.
4. Let batter rest for 5 to 10 minutes. This allows all of the ingredients to come together and gives the batter a better consistency.
5. Spray a non-stick skillet or griddle generously with vegetable oil and heat over medium heat.
6. Once the skillet is hot, add the batter using a ¼-cup measuring cup and pour the batter into the skillet to make the pancake. Use the measuring cup to help shape the pancake.
7. Cook until the sides appear set and bubbles form in the middle (about 2 to 3 minutes), then flip the pancake.
8. Once the pancake is cooked on that side, remove pancake from the heat and place on a plate.
9. Continue these steps with the rest of the batter. Serve with berries, if desired.

Protein 9 grams | Carbs 32 grams | Calories 269

3-INGREDIENT PANCAKES

MAKES 6 PANCAKES | SERVES 2

1 ripe banana, plus more for serving (optional)

2 large eggs
½ teaspoon baking powder

1. Add the banana to a bowl and mash it until it's nice and creamy—no lumps.
2. Crack the eggs into another bowl and whisk until they are thoroughly mixed.
3. Add the baking powder to the bowl of banana and then pour in the eggs. Whisk to completely combine everything together.
4. Spray a non-stick skillet or griddle generously with vegetable oil and heat over medium heat.
5. Once the skillet is hot, add 2 tablespoons of batter into the pan to make the pancake.
6. Cook until the sides appear set (you won't see any bubbles), then carefully flip the pancake.
7. Once the pancake is cooked on that side, remove the pancake from the heat and place on a plate.
8. Continue these steps with the rest of the batter. Serve with sliced banana, if desired.

Note:
These pancakes are pretty thin, they scrunch up easily, and they're a little difficult to flip. I used both a spatula and a fork to help flip them over and to remove them from the pan.

Protein 7 grams | Carbs 14 grams | Calories 123

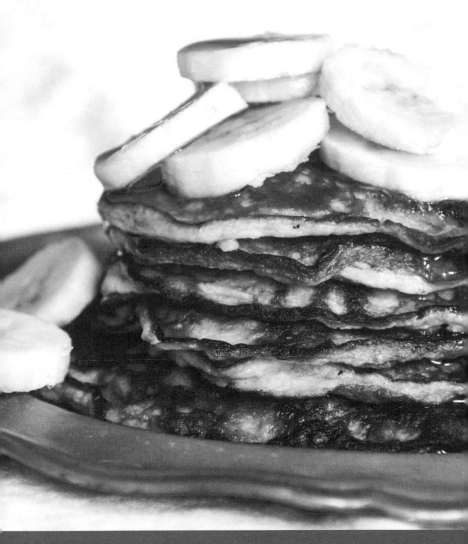

Three-Ingredient Pancakes are really a thing. All that stands between you and breakfast are three little ingredients that you probably have handy. These pancakes aren't the light and fluffy kind you're probably used to—they're super creamy and rich tasting. Because they're made with banana, eggs, and baking powder, they have a strong banana flavor. Want to tame that down a bit? Add some chocolate chips to the mix.

ALMOND BUTTER PANCAKES

MAKES 4 PANCAKES | SERVES 2

1 large egg
1 tablespoon coconut oil, melted
1 tablespoon maple syrup
1 tablespoon almond butter, plus more for serving

1 teaspoon baking powder
½ teaspoon vanilla extract
¼ teaspoon salt
½ cup 2% low-fat milk
¾ cup spelt flour
Cherries, for serving (optional)

1. In a large bowl, add the egg, coconut oil, maple syrup, almond butter, baking powder, vanilla, and salt, then whisk to thoroughly combine.
2. Add the milk to the mixture and whisk again to combine.
3. Add the flour to the mixture and whisk to thoroughly combine the ingredients.

Pancakes and weekends go together like silver and gold, and these golden pancakes are going to make your weekend great. They've got a subtle flavor from the almond butter inside the pancakes and a lot of nutty flavor from the almond butter poured over the top. These are a hardy, yet fluffy pancake that will keep you filled up until lunch.

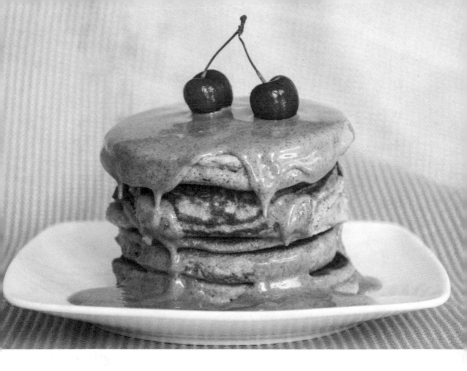

4. Let the batter rest for 2 to 3 minutes. This allows the batter to thicken up so that all the ingredients come together.
5. Spray a non-stick skillet or griddle generously with vegetable oil and heat over medium heat.
6. Once the skillet is hot, add the batter using a ¼-cup measuring cup and pour the batter into the skillet to make the pancake. Use the measuring cup to help shape the pancake.
7. Cook until the sides appear set and bubbles form in the middle (about 2 to 3 minutes), then flip the pancake.
8. Once the pancake is cooked on that side, remove pancake from the heat and place on a plate.
9. Continue these steps with the rest of the batter.
10. Serve pancakes with melted almond butter and cherries, if desired. To melt almond butter, scoop out desired amount into microwave-safe dish and heat on high in 30-second intervals until melted. Stir between heating.

Protein 13 grams | Carbs 38 grams | Calories 353

ALMOND BUTTER PANCAKES

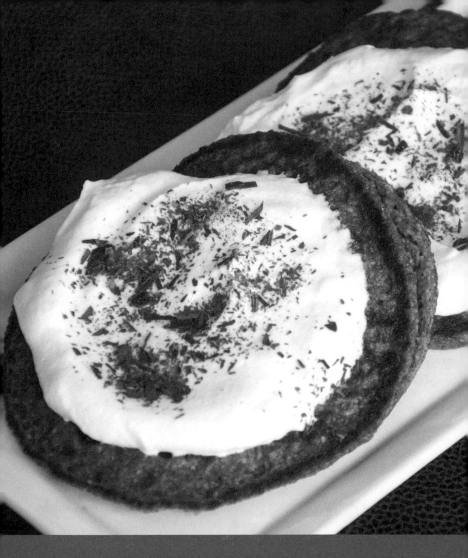

Combine coffee, chocolate, and cream and what do you get? That favorite Italian dessert tiramisu. Why not combine these same ingredients for some outrageously delicious, high-protein pancakes? These pancakes give you a hint of those three famous flavors in each and every bite. Top them with a bit of whipped cream and shaved chocolate for a decadent breakfast.

TIRAMISU PANCAKES

1¾ cups old-fashioned rolled oats
1½ tablespoons sugar-free
  vanilla Jell-O pudding mix
2 teaspoons instant espresso
1½ teaspoons cocoa powder
1½ teaspoons baking powder
1 teaspoon baking soda
½ teaspoon cinnamon

¼ teaspoon salt
2 tablespoons coconut oil, melted
1 tablespoon maple syrup
1 large egg
1 teaspoon vanilla extract
1 cup 2% low-fat milk
Whipped cream, for serving
Chocolate shavings, for serving

1. Add all of the ingredients, except for the whipped cream and chocolate shavings, to a blender. The melted coconut oil might harden up when combined with colder ingredients, so you can slightly warm the milk to help prevent this from happening if you'd like.
2. Blitz everything in the blender until you have a smooth liquid.
3. Pour the pancake mixture into a large bowl.
4. Let the batter rest for 2 to 3 minutes. This allows all of the ingredients to come together and gives the batter a better consistency.
5. Spray a non-stick skillet or griddle generously with vegetable oil and heat over medium heat.
6. Once the skillet is hot, add the batter using a ¼-cup measuring cup and pour the batter into the skillet to make the pancake. Use the measuring cup to help shape the pancake.
7. Cook until the sides appear set and bubbles form in the middle (about 2 to 3 minutes), then flip the pancake.
8. Once the pancake is cooked on that side, remove pancake from the heat and place on a plate.
9. Continue these steps with the rest of the batter.
10. Top with whipped cream and chocolate shavings.

Protein 8 grams | Carbs 28 grams | Calories 241

LEMON BLUEBERRY PANCAKES

MAKES 8 PANCAKES | SERVES 4

1½ cups spelt flour
1½ teaspoons baking powder
1 teaspoon baking soda
½ teaspoon salt
Zest from 1 lemon
2 tablespoons coconut oil, melted

2 large eggs, beaten
¼ cup 2% low-fat milk
¼ cup maple syrup, plus more for serving
1¼ cups plain kefir (slightly warmed)
½ cup blueberries

---

1. Add the flour, baking powder, baking soda, and salt to a large bowl and whisk to thoroughly combine.
2. Add the coconut oil, eggs, milk, maple syrup, lemon zest, and kefir to a bowl and whisk to combine. The melted coconut oil might harden up when combined with colder ingredients, so you can slightly warm the kefir to help prevent this from happening if you'd like.
3. Pour the wet ingredients into the dry ingredients and whisk to combine until all the ingredients are wet.
4. Let the batter rest for 2 to 3 minutes. This allows all of the ingredients to come together and gives the batter a better consistency.
5. Spray a non-stick skillet or griddle generously with vegetable oil and heat over medium heat.
6. Once the skillet is hot, add the batter using a ¼-cup measuring cup and pour the batter into the skillet to make the pancake. Use the measuring cup to help shape the pancake.
7. Place 3 to 5 blueberries onto each pancake. Keep the berries toward the center so it's easier to flip the pancake.

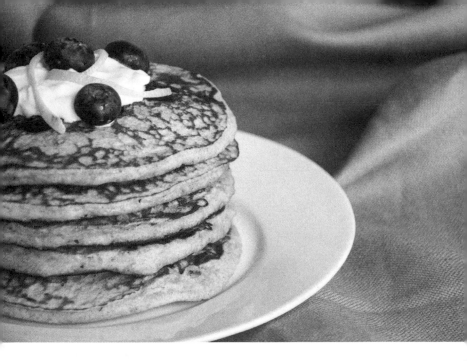

8. Cook until the sides appear set and bubbles form in the middle (about 2 to 3 minutes), then flip the pancake.
9. Once the pancake is cooked on that side, remove pancake from the heat and place on a plate.
10. Continue these steps with the rest of the batter. Serve with maple syrup.

Protein 13 grams | Carbs 50 grams | Calories 365

The tang of lemon with the mellow sweetness of blueberries is a match made in heaven. These pancakes combine the two flavors into what is sure to become a breakfast-time favorite. Since the kefir already has a bit of a tang to it, the lemon zest works really well with this batter. The addition of the blueberries makes these pancakes extra special. For a topping that is less sweet than maple syrup, try kefir, lemon zest, and blueberries.

LEMON BLUEBERRY PANCAKES

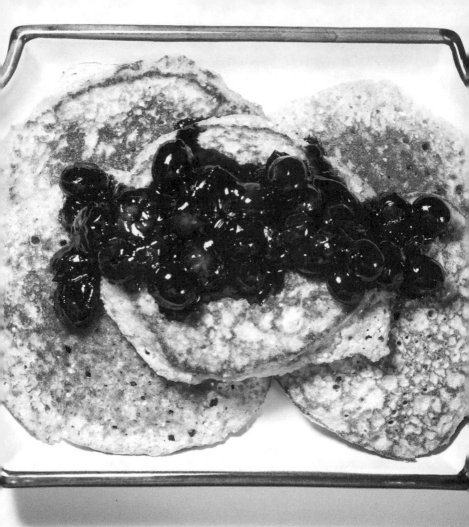

Quinoa isn't just a side dish to be served with beef or chicken. Include it in your pancakes for an extra dose of protein and fiber. It also adds a little crunch to your pancakes. These lightly sweetened pancakes weigh a little more than your traditional pancake but aren't heavy.

QUINOA PANCAKES

1 cup (any color) cooked quinoa
¾ cup quinoa flour
2 teaspoons baking powder
½ teaspoon salt
1 tablespoon melted butter
¼ cup Greek yogurt

2 tablespoons 2% low-fat milk
2 large eggs, beaten
2 tablespoons maple syrup
1 teaspoon vanilla extract
Fruit preserves, for serving
  (optional)

1. In a large bowl, add the quinoa, flour, baking powder, and salt together and whisk to thoroughly combine.
2. In another bowl, whisk butter, yogurt, milk, eggs, maple syrup, and vanilla. Whisk everything together so that it is well combined.
3. Add the wet ingredients to the dry ingredients and whisk until thoroughly combined.
4. Let the batter rest for 2 to 3 minutes. This allows all of the ingredients to come together and gives the batter a better consistency.
5. Spray a non-stick skillet or griddle generously with vegetable oil and heat over medium heat.
6. Once the skillet is hot, add the batter using a ¼-cup measuring cup and pour the batter into the skillet to make the pancake. Use the measuring cup to help shape the pancake.
7. Cook until the sides appear set and bubbles form in the middle (about 2 to 3 minutes), then flip the pancake.
8. Once the pancake is cooked on that side, remove pancake from the heat and place on a plate.
9. Continue these steps with the rest of the batter. Serve with fruit preserves, if desired.

Protein 10 grams | Carbs 31 grams | Calories 238

GREEK YOGURT OATMEAL PANCAKES

MAKES 8 PANCAKES | SERVES 4

1¾ cups old-fashioned rolled oats
1½ teaspoons baking powder
1 teaspoon baking soda
½ teaspoon cinnamon
¼ teaspoon salt
1 large egg

2 tablespoons coconut oil, melted
1 tablespoon maple syrup, plus more to serve
1 teaspoon vanilla extract
1 cup plain Greek yogurt
¼ cup 2% low-fat milk

1. Add all of the ingredients to a blender. The melted coconut oil might harden up when combined with colder ingredients, so you can slightly warm the milk to help prevent this from happening if you'd like.

These fluffy pancakes have a slightly tangy flavor due to the addition of Greek yogurt. They're also lightly sweetened with maple syrup. A stack of these pancakes is finished perfectly with an additional drizzle of maple syrup.

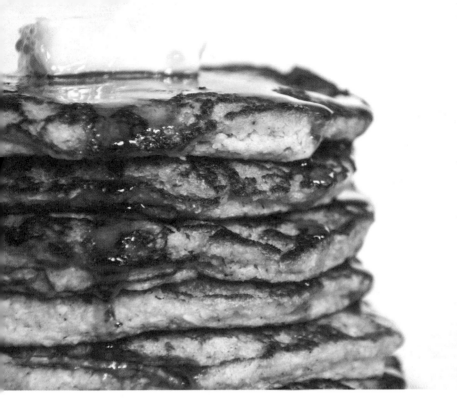

2. Blitz everything in the blender until you have a smooth liquid.
3. Pour the pancake mixture into a large bowl.
4. Let the batter rest for 5 to 10 minutes. This allows all of the ingredients to come together and gives the batter a better consistency.
5. Spray a non-stick skillet or griddle generously with vegetable oil and heat over medium heat.
6. Once the skillet is hot, add the batter using a ¼-cup measuring cup and pour the batter into the skillet to make the pancake. Use the measuring cup to help shape the pancake.
7. Cook until the sides appear set and bubbles form in the middle (about 2 minutes), then flip the pancake.
8. Once the pancake is cooked on that side, remove pancake from the heat and place on a plate.
9. Continue these steps with the rest of the batter. Serve with maple syrup.

Protein 11 grams | Carbs 30 grams | Calories 256 grams

GREEK YOGURT OATMEAL PANCAKES

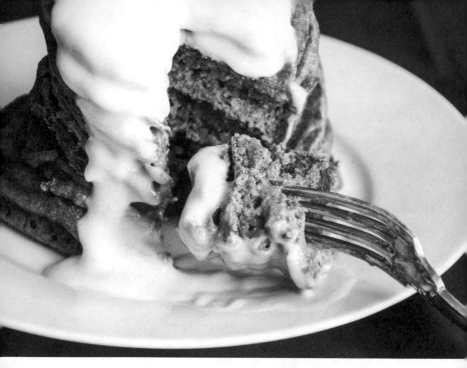

GINGERBREAD PANCAKES

MAKES 4 PANCAKES | SERVES 2

Topping

¼ cup plain Greek yogurt

1 tablespoon maple syrup

Pancakes

1 cup spelt flour

1 teaspoon baking soda

1 teaspoon ground ginger

1 teaspoon ground allspice

1 teaspoon cinnamon

¼ teaspoon ground cloves

¼ teaspoon salt

1 large egg

½ cup 2% low-fat milk

3 tablespoons maple syrup

1 teaspoon vanilla extract

For the Topping
1. Mix the Greek yogurt and maple syrup together until well combined and set aside.

For the Pancakes
1. In a large bowl, add the spelt flour, baking soda, ginger, allspice, cinnamon, cloves, and salt together and whisk to thoroughly combine.
2. In another bowl, whisk the egg, milk, maple syrup, and vanilla together until well combined.
3. Add the wet ingredients to the dry ingredients and whisk until thoroughly combined.
4. Let the batter rest for 2 to 3 minutes. This allows all of the ingredients to come together and gives the batter a better consistency.
5. Spray a non-stick skillet or griddle generously with vegetable oil and heat over medium heat.
6. Once the skillet is hot, add the batter using a ¼-cup measuring cup and pour the batter into the skillet to make the pancake. Use the measuring cup to help shape the pancake.
7. Cook until the sides appear set and bubbles form in the middle (about 2 to 3 minutes), then flip the pancake.
8. Once the pancake is cooked on that side, remove pancake from the heat and place on a plate.
9. Continue these steps with the rest of the batter. Serve with yogurt topping.

Protein 15 grams | Carbs 74 grams | Calories 422

These Gingerbread Pancakes are the perfect warm, comforting way to start those chilly winter mornings—and they'd be even better as a breakfast-in-bed treat. They're also great as a Christmas morning option, or for brinner (breakfast-for-dinner). They taste just like you're eating gingerbread cookies, complete with icing, but in a healthier pancake form.

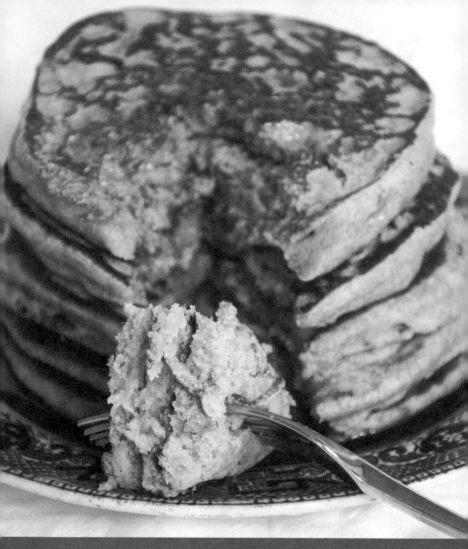

If you're looking for a good basic pancake recipe that looks great and tastes even better with maple syrup on top, then you need these Greek Yogurt Pancakes in your life. They're simple to throw together and have a ton of protein in them. So not only do they taste good, but they're good for you too. Simple perfection.

GREEK YOGURT PANCAKES

1 cup spelt flour
½ teaspoon baking powder
½ teaspoon baking soda
¾ cup plain Greek yogurt

½ cup + 2 tablespoons 2%
  low-fat milk
1 large egg
2 tablespoons maple syrup

1. Add the flour, baking powder, and baking soda to a bowl and whisk to combine.
2. In another bowl, whisk the yogurt, milk, egg, and maple syrup together until thoroughly combined.
3. Add the wet ingredients to the dry ingredients and whisk until thoroughly combined.
4. Let the batter rest for 2 to 3 minutes. This allows all of the ingredients to come together and gives the batter a better consistency.
5. Spray a non-stick skillet or griddle generously with vegetable oil and heat over medium heat.
6. Once the skillet is hot, add the batter using a ¼-cup measuring cup and pour the batter into the skillet to make the pancake. Use the measuring cup to help shape the pancake.
7. Cook until the sides appear set and bubbles form in the middle (about 2 to 3 minutes), then flip the pancake.
8. Once the pancake is cooked on that side, remove pancake from the heat and place on a plate.
9. Continue these steps with the rest of the batter.

Protein 10 grams | Carbs 32 grams | Calories 205

OATMEAL RAISIN COOKIE PANCAKES

MAKES 8 PANCAKES | SERVES 4

Topping

½ cup powdered sugar

1 tablespoon 2% low-fat milk

Pancakes

1¾ cups old-fashioned rolled oats

2 tablespoons brown sugar

1½ teaspoons baking powder

1 teaspoon baking soda

½ teaspoon cinnamon

¼ teaspoon salt

2 tablespoons coconut oil, melted

1 teaspoon vanilla extract

1 cup 2% low-fat milk

⅓ cup chopped golden raisins

For the Topping

1. In a small bowl, mix the powdered sugar and milk together until it's smooth. Set aside.

My favorite cookie is oatmeal raisin, so why not make it in pancake form? These pancakes taste just like you're biting into an oatmeal raisin cookie, but they're soft and fluffy. So why not have cookies (sort of) for breakfast?

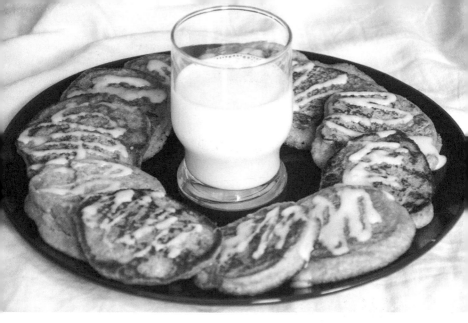

For the Pancakes

1. Add all of the ingredients, except for the raisins, to the blender. The melted coconut oil might harden up when combined with colder ingredients, so you can slightly warm the milk to help prevent this from happening if you'd like.
2. Blitz everything in the blender until you have a smooth liquid.
3. Pour the pancake mixture into a large bowl.
4. Stir in the chopped raisins.
5. Let the batter rest for 5 to 10 minutes. This allows all of the ingredients to come together and gives the batter a better consistency.
6. Spray a non-stick skillet or griddle generously with vegetable oil and heat over medium heat.
7. Once the skillet is hot, add the batter using a ¼-cup measuring cup and pour the batter into the skillet to make the pancake. Use the measuring cup to help shape the pancake.
8. Cook until the sides appear set and bubbles form in the middle (about 2 to 3 minutes), then flip the pancake.
9. Once the pancake is cooked on that side, remove pancake from the heat and place on a plate.
10. Continue these steps with the rest of the batter.
11. Top with sugar topping.

Protein 8 grams | Carbs 50 grams | Calories 315

OATMEAL RAISIN COOKIE PANCAKES

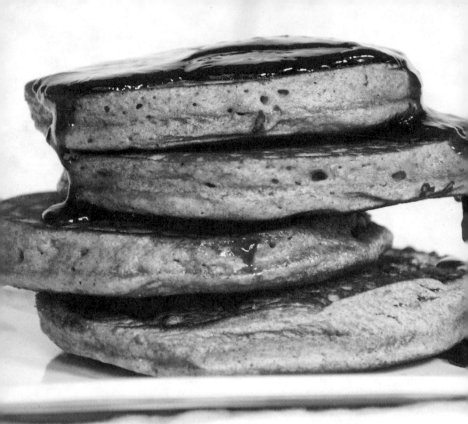

PEANUT BUTTER AND JELLY PANCAKES

MAKES 8 PANCAKES | SERVES 4

1½ cups spelt flour
¾ cup powdered peanut butter
1½ teaspoons baking powder
1 teaspoon baking soda
½ teaspoon salt

2 large eggs, beaten
1 tablespoon butter, melted
1½ cups 2% low-fat milk
Concord grape jelly, for serving

1. Add flour, powdered peanut butter, baking powder, baking soda, and salt to a bowl and whisk to combine.
2. In another bowl, whisk the eggs, butter, and milk together until thoroughly combined.
3. Add the wet ingredients to the dry ingredients and whisk until thoroughly combined.
4. Let the batter rest for 2 to 3 minutes. This allows all of the ingredients to come together and gives the batter a better consistency.
5. Spray a non-stick skillet or griddle generously with vegetable oil and heat over medium heat.
6. Once the skillet is hot, add the batter using a ¼-cup measuring cup and pour the batter into the skillet to make the pancake. Use the measuring cup to help shape the pancake.
7. Cook until the sides appear set and bubbles form in the middle (about 2 to 3 minutes), then flip the pancake.
8. Once the pancake is cooked on that side, remove pancake from the heat and place on a plate.
9. Continue these steps with the rest of the batter. Top with the grape jelly.

Note:
For the topping, I melted ¼ cup Concord grape jelly in the microwave, and then drizzled it over the pancakes right before serving.

Protein 16 grams | Carbs 41 grams | Calories 320

Peanut butter and jelly sandwiches aren't just for lunch or kids anymore. Nope. How about Peanut Butter and Jelly Pancakes for breakfast? These pancakes are filled with peanut buttery goodness and topped off with classic grape jelly. They might just be the perfect thing for dinner too.

BACON PANCAKES

8 slices center-cut bacon
1½ cups spelt flour
1½ teaspoons baking powder
1 teaspoon baking soda
½ teaspoon salt
2 large eggs, beaten

1 tablespoon butter, melted
1 teaspoon vanilla extract
1¼ cups 2% low-fat milk
¼ cup maple syrup

1. Preheat the oven to 350°F.
2. Arrange the bacon, in a single layer, on a rimmed baking sheet lined with parchment paper. This makes cleanup a whole lot easier.
3. Slide the bacon into the oven and cook for 30 minutes, or until the bacon is done.
4. Remove the bacon from the oven and place the bacon on a paper towel-lined plate to cool.
5. In a large bowl, add the flour, baking powder, baking soda, and salt. Whisk to combine ingredients.
6. In another bowl, add the eggs, butter, vanilla, milk, and maple syrup and whisk to combine ingredients.
7. Add the wet ingredients to the dry ingredients and whisk to thoroughly combine everything.
8. Let the batter rest for 2 to 3 minutes. This allows all of the ingredients to come together and gives the batter a better consistency.
9. Spray a non-stick skillet or griddle generously with vegetable oil and heat over medium heat.
10. Once the skillet is hot, place a bacon strip onto the skillet. Pour ¼ cup of batter on top of the bacon. Spread the batter evenly over the bacon, as well as the sides of the bacon.

Continued

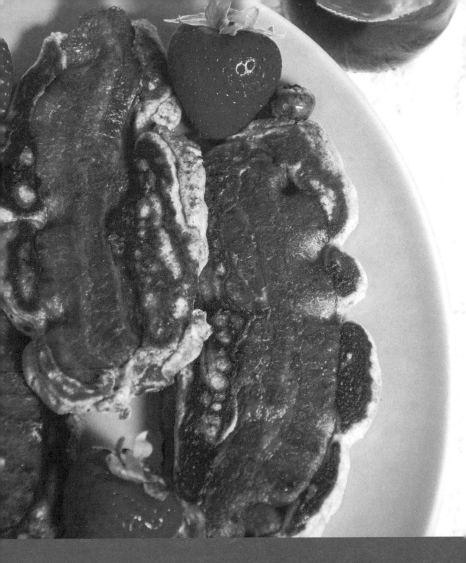

How do you make a breakfast even more perfect? Add bacon! And because the bacon is in the pancakes, it leaves more room on your plate for even more pancakes. These Bacon Pancakes are the best of all worlds . . . tastes of salt, sweet, and a bit of fat in every bite. In other words . . . heaven on a plate.

11. Cook until the sides appear set, then flip the pancake over to cook. You may notice that these pancakes cook a little quicker on the bacon side.
12. Once the pancake is cooked on that side, remove the pancake from the heat and place on a plate.
13. Continue these steps with the rest of the batter.

Protein 18 grams | Carbs 38 grams | Calories 368

RASPBERRY ALMOND PANCAKES

MAKES 4 PANCAKES | SERVES 2

Raspberry Topping

1½ cups frozen raspberries, thawed

2 tablespoons honey

Pancakes

1½ cups almond flour
1 teaspoon baking powder
¼ teaspoon salt
¼ teaspoon cinnamon

2 large eggs, beaten
¼ cup 2% low-fat milk
1 tablespoon maple syrup
1 teaspoon vanilla extract

Light, fluffy, and fruity—that's what these pancakes are. Raspberries and almonds go together perfectly, and in a pancake they are exactly what you want for breakfast. With the maple syrup in the pancakes and the raspberries in and on top of the pancakes, the end result is a subtly sweet, slightly tart breakfast.

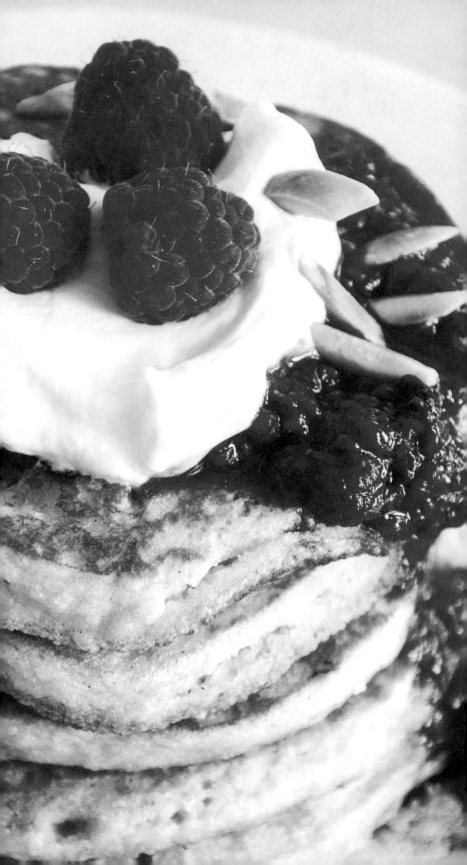

For the Raspberry Topping

1. Mix the raspberries with the honey. While mixing the fruit, also smash it to extract more liquid.
2. Pour the Raspberry Topping into a sandwich bag, seal, and set aside.

For the Pancakes

1. Add the flour, baking powder, salt, and cinnamon to a bowl and whisk to thoroughly combine.
2. In a separate bowl, whisk the remaining ingredients together.
3. Add the wet ingredients to the dry ingredients and whisk to thoroughly combine them.
4. Let the batter rest for 5 to 10 minutes. This allows all of the ingredients to come together and gives the batter a better consistency.
5. Spray a non-stick skillet or griddle generously with vegetable oil and heat over medium-high heat.
6. Once the skillet is hot, add batter using a ¼-cup measuring cup and pour the batter into the skillet to make the pancake. Gently spread the batter into a round shape with the measuring cup.
7. Snip one corner of the bag containing the Raspberry Topping and drizzle some of it over the top of the pancake. Use a toothpick to drag the raspberries through the pancake base.
8. Cook until the sides appear set and bubbles form in the middle (about 2 to 3 minutes), then flip the pancake.
9. Once the pancake is cooked on that side, remove pancake from the heat and place on a plate.
10. Continue these steps with the rest of the batter.
11. Top with the remaining raspberry topping.

Protein 20 grams | Carbs 47 grams | Calories 602

RASPBERRY ALMOND PANCAKES

PEANUT, BANANA, AND CHOCOLATE PANCAKES

MAKES 8 PANCAKES | SERVES 4

1 cup spelt flour
¼ cup powdered peanut butter
½ teaspoon baking powder
½ teaspoon baking soda
¾ cup plain Greek yogurt
1 ripe medium banana, mashed, plus more for serving (optional)

¼ cup + 2 tablespoons 2% low-fat milk
1 large egg
2 tablespoons maple syrup
½ cup chocolate chips, plus more for serving (optional)
Peanut butter, for serving (optional)

1. Add the flour, powdered peanut butter, baking powder, and baking soda to a bowl and whisk to combine.
2. In another bowl, whisk the yogurt, mashed banana, milk, egg, and maple syrup until combined.
3. Add the wet ingredients to the dry ingredients and whisk until thoroughly combined.
4. Stir in the chocolate chips.
5. Let the batter rest for 2 to 3 minutes. This allows all of the ingredients to come together and gives the batter a better consistency.
6. Spray a non-stick skillet or griddle generously with vegetable oil and heat over medium heat.
7. Once the skillet is hot, add the batter using a ¼-cup measuring cup and pour the batter into the skillet to make the pancake. Use the measuring cup to help shape the pancake.

Continued

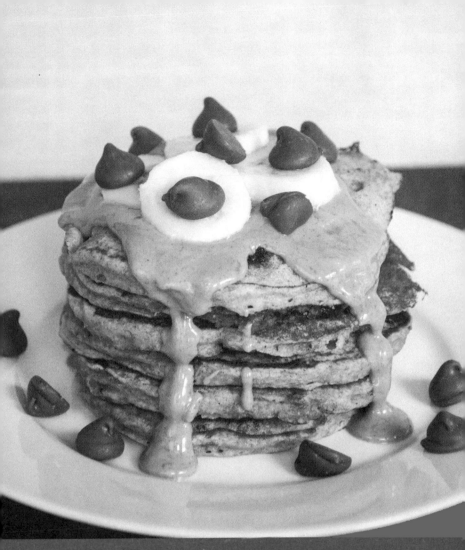

These pancakes are a dream come true for peanut butter lovers. Using powdered peanut butter gives you all that great peanut butter flavor (and protein) without all the added fat. Throw in the sweetness from the bananas and those chocolatey chocolate chips and you've got what might be the perfect pancake.

8. Cook until the sides appear set and bubbles form in the middle (about 2 to 3 minutes), then flip the pancake.
9. Once the pancake is cooked on that side, remove pancake from the heat and place on a plate.
10. Continue these steps with the rest of the batter.
11. If desired, top with melted peanut butter, sliced banana, and chocolate chips.

Protein 11 grams | Carbs 44 grams | Calories 292

HIGH-PROTEIN PANCAKES

VANILLA COCONUT PANCAKES

MAKES 8 PANCAKES | SERVES 4

Vanilla Coconut Topping

1 cup canned full-fat coconut milk

¼ cup maple syrup

1½ teaspoons vanilla extract

Small pinch salt

Pancakes

1½ cups spelt flour

¼ cup shredded unsweetened coconut, toasted (plus more for serving)

1½ teaspoons baking powder

1 teaspoon baking soda

½ teaspoon salt

2 large eggs, beaten

2 tablespoons coconut oil, melted

1 tablespoon vanilla extract

¼ cup maple syrup

¼ cup canned full-fat coconut milk

1¼ cups plain kefir

These pancakes are what weekend breakfasts are all about: a light and fluffy pancake, slightly sweet and incredibly delicious. To add to the flavor of the pancakes, the vanilla coconut topping brings the flavors together even more.

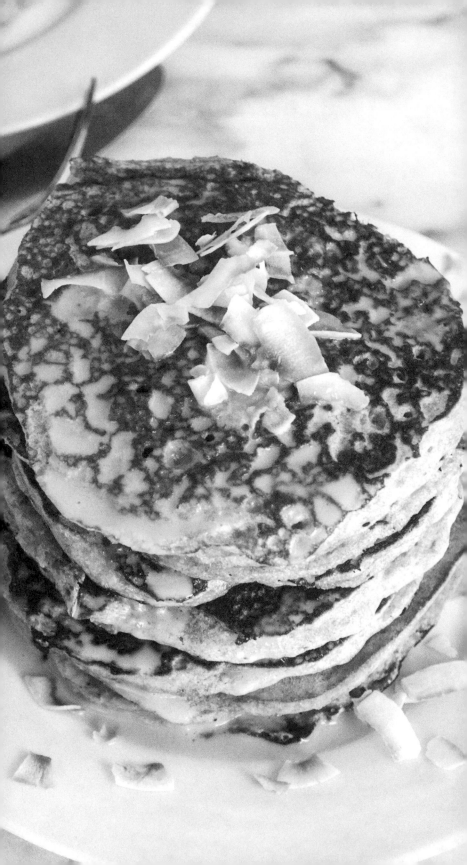

For the Vanilla Coconut Topping

1. Add all the ingredients to a small saucepan and heat over medium heat.
2. Whisk occasionally and cook until the mixture begins to thicken (approximately 7 minutes).
3. Remove from the heat to let it cool slightly.

For the Pancakes

1. In a large bowl, add the flour, coconut, baking powder, baking soda, and salt. Whisk to combine ingredients.
2. In another bowl, add the eggs, coconut oil, vanilla, maple syrup, coconut milk, and kefir and whisk to combine ingredients. The melted coconut oil might harden up when combined with colder ingredients, so you can slightly warm the kefir to help prevent this from happening if you'd like.
3. Add the wet ingredients to the dry ingredients and whisk to thoroughly combine everything.
4. Let the batter rest for 2 to 3 minutes. This allows all of the ingredients to come together and gives the batter a better consistency.
5. Spray a non-stick skillet or griddle generously with vegetable oil and heat over medium heat.
6. Once the skillet is hot, add the batter using a ¼-cup measuring cup and pour the batter into the skillet to make the pancake. Use the measuring cup to help shape the pancake.
7. Cook until the sides appear set and bubbles form in the middle (about 2 to 3 minutes), then flip the pancake.
8. Once the pancake is cooked on that side, remove pancake from the heat and place on a plate.
9. Continue these steps with the rest of the batter.
10. Spoon the Vanilla Coconut Topping over the pancakes and sprinkle with the toasted coconut before serving.

Note:

To toast the coconut, toss it into a skillet and heat over medium heat. Continue to stir the coconut as it heats and turn the flakes over so that they get toasted on both sides. Continue doing this until most of the coconut is golden brown.

Protein 13 grams | Carbs 48 grams | Calories 399

CHOCOLATE COCONUT ALMOND PANCAKES

1½ cups almond flour
½ cup shredded, unsweetened coconut, toasted
1 teaspoon baking powder
1 teaspoon baking soda
¼ teaspoon salt
2 large eggs, beaten
½ cup canned full-fat coconut milk

1 tablespoon maple syrup, plus more for serving
1 teaspoon vanilla extract
½ cup chocolate chips
Toasted coconut, roasted almonds, and shaved chocolate, for serving

1. Add the flour, shredded coconut, baking powder, baking soda, and salt to a bowl and whisk to thoroughly combine.
2. In a separate bowl, whisk the eggs, coconut milk, maple syrup, and vanilla together.
3. Add the wet ingredients to the dry ingredients and whisk to thoroughly combine them.

If you love Almond Joy candy bars, you're going to love starting your day off with these Coconut Almond Pancakes. They're loaded with coconut, almonds, and chocolate. The almond flour makes them slightly denser than a pancake made with regular flour, but they're not heavy. Top them off with toasted coconut, roasted almonds, shaved chocolate, and a touch of maple syrup for a heavenly breakfast treat.

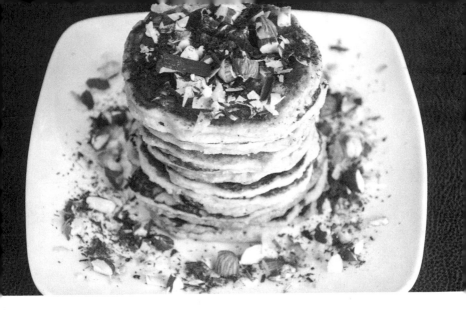

4. Stir in the chocolate chips.
5. Let the batter rest for 5 to 10 minutes. This allows all of the ingredients to come together and gives the batter a better consistency.
6. Spray a non-stick skillet or griddle generously with vegetable oil and heat over medium heat.
7. Once the skillet is hot, add the batter using a ¼-cup measuring cup and pour the batter into the skillet to make the pancake. Use the measuring cup to help shape the pancake.
8. Cook until the sides appear set and bubbles form in the middle (about 2 to 3 minutes), then flip the pancake.
9. Once the pancake is cooked on that side, remove pancake from the heat and place on a plate.
10. Continue these steps with the rest of the batter.
11. Top with toasted coconut, roasted almonds, shredded chocolate, and a drizzle more of maple syrup, if you'd like.

Note:
These pancakes cook better if they're made smaller than the usual ¼-cup-size pancake. You can make them bigger, but they just get a little more difficult to flip. To toast the coconut, toss it into a skillet and heat over medium heat. Continue to stir the coconut as it heats and turn the flakes over so that they get toasted on both sides. Continue doing this until most of the coconut is golden brown.

Protein 13 grams | Carbs 23 grams | Calories 462

CHOCOLATE COCONUT ALMOND PANCAKES

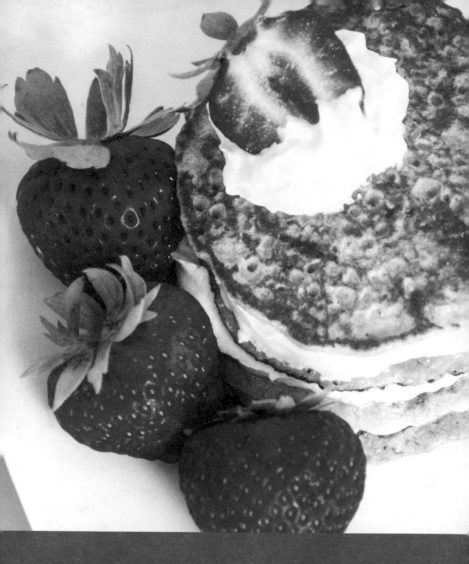

Strawberry shortcake is the perfect dessert when strawberries are at their peak, so why not turn that scrumptious treat into a delicious breakfast? Layer each pancake with a bit of whipped cream for that true strawberry shortcake taste!

STRAWBERRY SHORTCAKE PANCAKES

1¾ cups old-fashioned rolled oats
1½ teaspoons baking powder
1 teaspoon baking soda
½ teaspoon cinnamon
¼ teaspoon salt
2 tablespoons coconut oil, melted

1 tablespoon maple syrup
1 large egg
1 teaspoon vanilla extract
1½ cups 2% low-fat milk
1 cup thinly sliced strawberries
Whipped cream and strawberries, to serve

---

1. Add all of the ingredients, except for the strawberries, to a blender. The melted coconut oil might harden up when combined with colder ingredients, so you can slightly warm the milk to help prevent this from happening if you'd like.
2. Blitz everything in the blender until you have a smooth liquid.
3. Pour the pancake mixture into a large bowl.
4. Let the batter rest for 5 to 10 minutes. This allows all of the ingredients to come together and gives the batter a better consistency.
5. Spray a non-stick skillet or griddle generously with vegetable oil and heat over medium heat.

Continued

6. Once the skillet is hot, add the batter using a ¼-cup measuring cup and pour the batter into the skillet to make the pancake. Use the measuring cup to help shape the pancake. Place the sliced strawberries in a single layer in the batter.
7. Cook until the sides appear set and bubbles form in the middle (about 2 minutes), then flip the pancake. You may need to let these cook a little longer on the first side so that they don't fall apart when you flip them. The strawberries are heavy and can cause these pancakes to break if they're not completely set on the first side.
8. Once the pancake is cooked on that side, remove pancake from the heat and place on a plate.
9. Continue these steps with the rest of the batter.
10. To serve, layer pancakes with whipped cream and top with strawberries.

Protein 10 grams | Carbs 36 grams | Calories 283

HIGH-PROTEIN PANCAKES

PEANUT BUTTER CUP PANCAKES

1¾ cups old-fashioned rolled oats
¼ cup powdered peanut butter
1½ teaspoons baking powder
1 teaspoon baking soda
½ teaspoon cinnamon
¼ teaspoon salt

2 tablespoons coconut oil, melted
1 tablespoon maple syrup
1 large egg
1 teaspoon vanilla extract
1½ cups 2% low-fat milk
½ cup chocolate chips

1. Add all of the ingredients, except for the chocolate chips, to a blender. The melted coconut oil might harden up when combined with colder ingredients, so you can slightly warm the milk to help prevent this from happening if you'd like.

Continued

Peanut butter and chocolate are time-proven complements. These pancakes combine both for a not-too-sweet-but-oh-so-delicious breakfast treat. Powdered peanut butter is the secret ingredient that gives you that great peanutty flavor in these pancakes. Top this delicious stack of pancakes with some melted peanut butter and chocolate syrup for a slightly sinful treat.

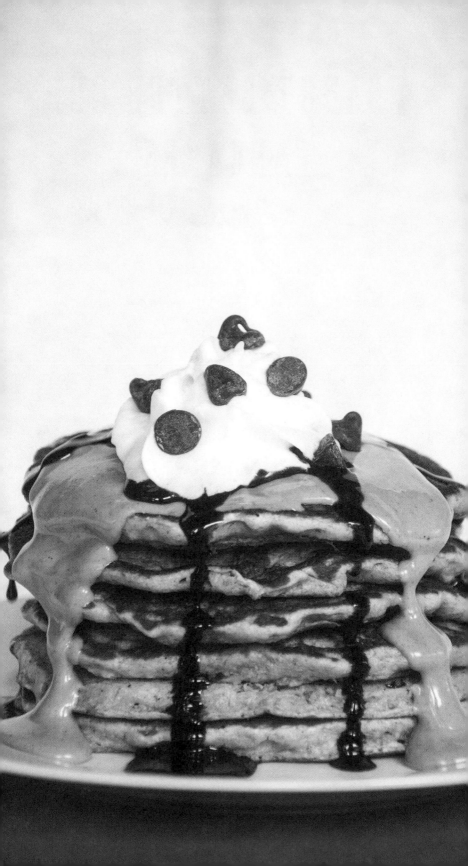

2. Blitz everything in the blender until you have a smooth liquid.
3. Pour the pancake batter into a large bowl.
4. Stir in the chocolate chips.
5. Let the batter rest for 5 to 10 minutes. This allows all of the ingredients to come together and gives the batter a better consistency.
6. Spray a non-stick skillet or griddle generously with vegetable oil and heat over medium heat.
7. Once the skillet is hot, add the batter using a ¼-cup measuring cup and pour the batter into the skillet to make the pancake. Use the measuring cup to help shape the pancake.
8. Cook until the sides appear set and bubbles form in the middle (about 2 to 3 minutes), then flip the pancake.
9. Once the pancake is cooked on that side, remove pancake from the heat and placc on a plate.
10. Continue these steps with the rest of the batter.

Protein 11 grams | Carbs 42 grams | Calories 351

MEXICAN CHOCOLATE PANCAKES

MAKES 8 PANCAKES | SERVES 4

1 cup spelt flour
¼ cup unsweetened cocoa
1 teaspoon cinnamon
½ teaspoon baking powder
½ teaspoon baking soda

¾ cup plain Greek yogurt
¼ cup + 2 tablespoons
   2% low-fat milk
1 large egg
2 tablespoons maple syrup

1. Add the flour, cocoa, cinnamon, baking powder, and baking soda to a bowl and whisk to combine.
2. In another bowl, whisk the yogurt, milk, egg, and maple syrup together until thoroughly combined.
3. Add the wet ingredients to the dry ingredients and whisk until thoroughly combined.
4. Let the batter rest for 2 to 3 minutes. This allows all of the ingredients to come together and gives the batter a better consistency.
5. Spray a non-stick skillet or griddle generously with vegetable oil and heat over medium heat.
6. Once the skillet is hot, add the batter using a ¼-cup measuring cup and pour the batter into the skillet to make the pancake. Use the measuring cup to help shape the pancake.
7. Cook until the sides appear set and bubbles form in the middle (about 2 to 3 minutes), then flip the pancake.
8. Once the pancake is cooked on that side, remove pancake from the heat and place on a plate.
9. Continue these steps with the rest of the batter.

Protein 11 grams | Carbs 34 grams | Calories 207

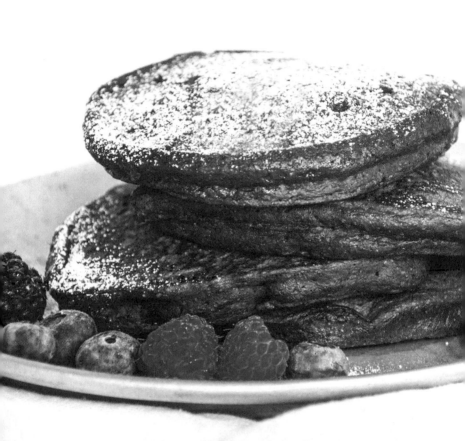

The rich flavor of chocolate combines with the heady flavor and aroma of cinnamon to make these Mexican Chocolate Pancakes the perfect morning starter. Your kitchen will be filled with the scent of chocolate and cinnamon as you make these rich pancakes. Top with powdered sugar and serve with fresh berries for an extra special breakfast.

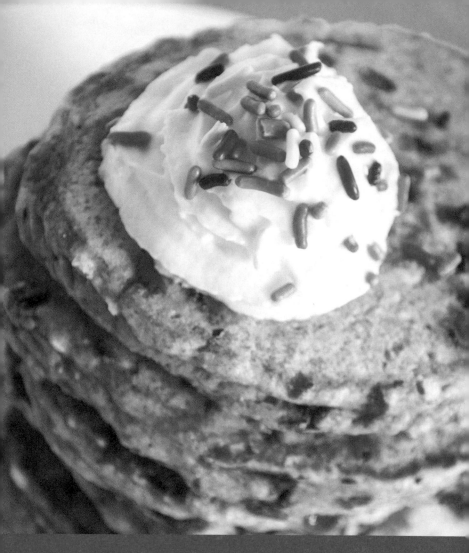

What's more fun than sprinkles? Pancakes filled with sprinkles! These pancakes are the perfect way to celebrate that special someone's birthday. The vanilla pudding makes them taste just like a vanilla birthday cake. A big dollop of whipped cream is the perfect way to set off a stack of these pretty birthday pancakes.

BIRTHDAY SURPRISE PANCAKES

MAKES 8 PANCAKES | SERVES 4

1 cup spelt flour
2 tablespoons sugar-free vanilla
  pudding mix
½ teaspoon baking powder
½ teaspoon baking soda
¾ cup plain Greek yogurt

½ cup + 2 tablespoons
  2% low-fat milk
1 large egg
2 tablespoons maple syrup
¼ cup rainbow sprinkles, plus
  more for topping (optional)

1. Add the flour, pudding, baking powder, and baking soda to a bowl and whisk to combine.
2. In another bowl, whisk the yogurt, milk, egg, and maple syrup together until thoroughly combined.
3. Add the wet ingredients to the dry ingredients and whisk until thoroughly combined.
4. Let the batter rest for 2 to 3 minutes. This allows all of the ingredients to come together and gives the batter a better consistency.
5. After the batter rests, stir in the sprinkles.
6. Spray a non-stick skillet or griddle generously with vegetable oil and heat over medium heat.
7. Once the skillet is hot, add the batter using a ¼-cup measuring cup and pour the batter into the skillet to make the pancake. Use the measuring cup to help shape the pancake.
8. Cook until the sides appear set and bubbles form in the middle (about 2 to 3 minutes), then flip the pancake.
9. Once the pancake is cooked on that side, remove pancake from the heat and place on a plate.
10. Continue these steps with the rest of the batter.

Protein 10 grams | Carbs 32 grams | Calories 205

GREEN MONSTER PANCAKES

1½ cups spelt flour
2 tablespoons hemp powder
1 tablespoon spirulina powder
1½ teaspoons baking powder
1 teaspoon baking soda
½ teaspoon salt
2 tablespoons coconut oil, melted

1½ tablespoons honey
1 tablespoon vanilla extract
2 large eggs, beaten
¼ cup canned full-fat coconut milk
1¼ cups plain kefir (slightly warmed)

1. Add the spelt flour, hemp powder, spirulina powder, baking powder, baking soda, and salt to a bowl and whisk to combine.
2. In another bowl, whisk the coconut oil, honey, vanilla, eggs, coconut milk, and kefir together until they are well combined. The melted coconut oil might harden up when combined with colder ingredients, so you can slightly warm the kefir to help prevent this from happening if you'd like.
3. Add the wet ingredients to the dry ingredients and whisk together until thoroughly combined.
4. Let the batter rest for 2 to 3 minutes. This allows all of the ingredients to come together and gives the batter a better consistency.
5. Spray a non-stick skillet or griddle generously with vegetable oil and heat over medium heat.
6. Once the skillet is hot, add the batter using a ¼-cup measuring cup and pour the batter into the skillet

to make the pancake. Use the measuring cup to help shape the pancake.

7. Cook until the sides appear set and bubbles form in the middle (about 2 to 3 minutes), then flip the pancake.
8. Once the pancake is cooked on that side, remove pancake from the heat and place on a plate.
9. Continue these steps with the rest of the batter.

Protein 15 grams | Carbs 45 grams | Calories 386

How about an extra boost of protein and vital nutrients? These Green Monster Pancakes are green because of the addition of spirulina and hemp powder. Instead of drinking your greens, you can eat them in these pancakes. These taste great topped with strawberries and drizzled with maple syrup or a little chocolate.

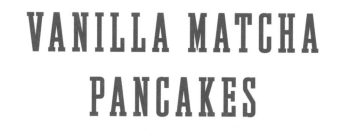

VANILLA MATCHA PANCAKES

1¾ cups old-fashioned rolled oats

2 tablespoons unsweetened matcha powder

2 tablespoons sugar-free vanilla pudding mix

1½ teaspoons baking powder

1 teaspoon baking soda

¼ teaspoon salt

2 tablespoons coconut oil, melted

1 tablespoon maple syrup

1 large egg

1 teaspoon vanilla extract

1½ cups 2% low-fat milk

1. Add all of the ingredients to a blender. The melted coconut oil might harden up when combined with colder ingredients, so you can slightly warm the milk to help prevent this from happening if you'd like.
2. Blitz everything in the blender until you have a smooth liquid.
3. Pour the pancake mixture into a large bowl.
4. Let the batter rest for 5 to 10 minutes. This allows all of the ingredients to come together and gives the batter a better consistency.
5. Spray a non-stick skillet or griddle generously with vegetable oil and heat over medium heat.
6. Once the skillet is hot, add the batter using a ¼-cup measuring cup and pour the batter into the skillet to make the pancake. Use the measuring cup to help shape the pancake.
7. Cook until the sides appear set and bubbles form in the middle (about 2 to 3 minutes), then flip the pancake.
8. Once the pancake is cooked on that side, remove pancake from the heat and place on a plate.
9. Continue these steps with the rest of the batter.

Protein 9 grams | Carbs 36 grams | Calories 294

These protein pancakes come with an extra bonus of antioxidants from the matcha (green tea) powder. Their crisp outside and fluffy insides are flavored with the matcha and just a hint of vanilla. These not-too-sweet pancakes are perfect when topped with a drizzle of maple syrup or a simple sprinkling of powdered sugar.

PIÑA COLADA PANCAKES

MAKES 8 PANCAKES | SERVES 4

1 cup spelt flour
½ teaspoon baking powder
½ teaspoon baking soda
¾ cup plain Greek yogurt
½ cup + 2 tablespoons canned full-fat coconut milk

1 large egg
2 tablespoons maple syrup
1 teaspoon vanilla extract
½ cup finely diced pineapple (if using canned pineapple, be sure to drain excess liquid)

1. Add the flour, baking powder, and baking soda to a bowl and whisk to combine.
2. In another bowl, whisk the yogurt, coconut milk, egg, maple syrup, and vanilla together until thoroughly combined.
3. Add the wet ingredients to the dry ingredients and whisk together until thoroughly combined.
4. Once everything is mixed together, stir in the pineapple.
5. Let the batter rest for 2 to 3 minutes. This allows all of the ingredients to come together and gives the batter a better consistency.
6. Spray a non-stick skillet or griddle generously with vegetable oil and heat over medium heat.
7. Once the skillet is hot, add the batter using a ¼-cup measuring cup and pour the batter into the skillet to make the pancake. Use the measuring cup to help shape the pancake.
8. Cook until the sides appear set and bubbles form in the middle (about 2 to 3 minutes), then flip the pancake.
9. Once the pancake is cooked on that side, remove pancake from the heat and place on a plate.
10. Continue these steps with the rest of the batter.

Protein 9 grams | Carbs 33 grams | Calories 260

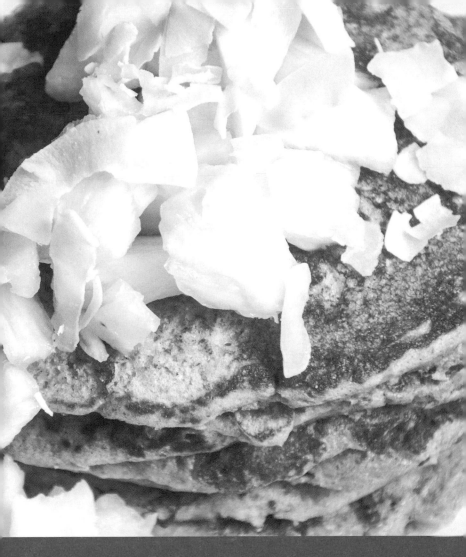

All the flavors of a piña colada cocktail can be in your morning pancake (these also make for a great brinner [breakfast-for-dinner], by the way). You can use fresh or canned pineapple in these—just make sure you drain the liquid if you use the canned pineapple. Top these off with more fresh pineapple and coconut.

PIÑA COLADA PANCAKES

CHERRY ALMOND PANCAKES

1½ cups almond flour
1 teaspoon baking powder
1 teaspoon baking soda
¼ teaspoon salt
2 large eggs, beaten
1 tablespoon maple syrup

1 teaspoon vanilla extract
½ cup canned full-fat coconut
  milk
½ cup finely diced sweet
  cherries
¼ cup sliced almonds

1. Add the flour, baking powder, baking soda, and salt to a bowl and whisk to thoroughly combine.
2. In a separate bowl, whisk the eggs, maple syrup, vanilla, and coconut milk together.
3. Add the wet ingredients to the dry ingredients and whisk to thoroughly combine them.

These Cherry Almond Pancakes are a dream. They have bits of sweet cherry in every bite and a great almond flavor. Not only do they have a crisp exterior, they get additional crunch from the sliced almonds. Top these with more cherries, and you've got yourself a very special, protein-filled breakfast.

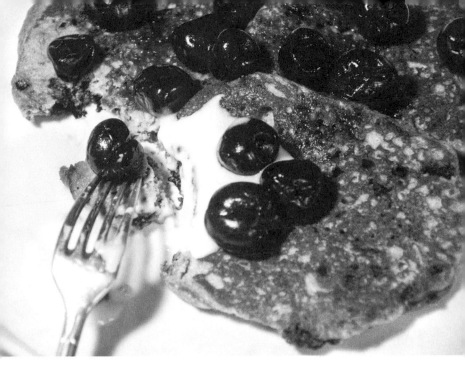

4. Now whisk in the cherries and almonds and mix until everything is well blended.
5. Let the batter rest for 5 to 10 minutes. This allows all of the ingredients to come together and gives the batter a better consistency.
6. Spray a non-stick skillet or griddle generously with vegetable oil and heat over medium-high heat.
7. Once the skillet is hot, add the batter using a ¼-cup measuring cup and pour the batter into the skillet to make the pancake. Use the measuring cup to help shape the pancake.
8. Cook until the sides appear set and bubbles form in the middle (about 2 to 3 minutes), then flip the pancake.
9. Once the pancake is cooked on that side, remove pancake from the heat and place on a plate.
10. Continue these steps with the rest of the batter.

Protein 14 grams | Carbs 18 grams | Calories 400

CHERRY ALMOND PANCAKES

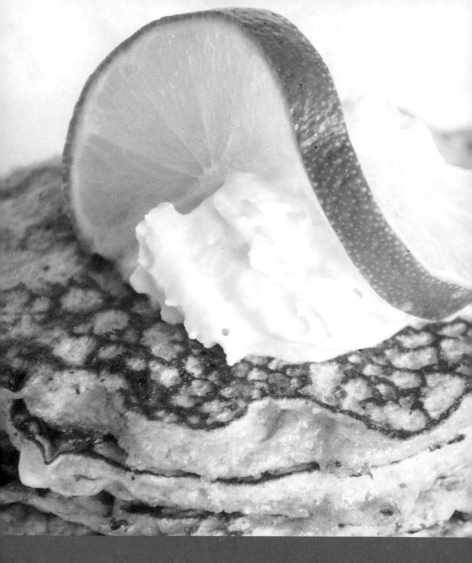

Key lime pie is so refreshing on a hot summer day. Why not enjoy these key lime pancakes for your summer breakfast? Not only are they packed with protein, they're packed with lime flavor. It makes you feel like you're eating pie for breakfast, especially when topped with whipped cream.

KEY LIME PANCAKES

2 eggs
½ cup cottage cheese
½ teaspoon vanilla extract
1 tablespoon honey
Zest from 1 lime

¼ cup spelt flour
½ teaspoon baking powder
¼ teaspoon baking soda
2 teaspoons sugar-free lime
    Jell-O mix

1. Whisk the eggs, cottage cheese, vanilla, honey, and lime zest together and set aside.
2. In another bowl, whisk the remaining ingredients together until well combined.
3. Add the wet ingredients to the dry ingredients and whisk until thoroughly combined.
4. Spray a non-stick skillet or griddle generously with vegetable oil and heat over medium heat.
5. Once the skillet is hot, add the batter using a ¼-cup measuring cup and pour the batter into the skillet to make the pancake. Use the measuring cup to help shape the pancake.
6. Cook until the sides appear set and bubbles form in the middle (about 2 to 3 minutes), then flip the pancake.
7. Once the pancake is cooked on that side, remove pancake from the heat and place on a plate.
8. Continue these steps with the rest of the batter.

Protein 15 grams | Carbs 22 grams | Calories 211

PUMPKIN SPICE PANCAKES

MAKES 8 PANCAKES | SERVES 4

1½ cups old-fashioned rolled oats
1½ teaspoons baking powder
½ teaspoon baking soda
½ teaspoon cinnamon
½ teaspoon ground allspice
½ teaspoon ground ginger
¼ teaspoon salt

½ cup canned pumpkin
2 tablespoons coconut oil, melted
2 tablespoons maple syrup
1 large egg
1 teaspoon vanilla extract
1 cup 2% low-fat milk

1. Add all of the ingredients to a blender. The melted coconut oil might harden up when combined with colder ingredients, so you can slightly warm the milk to help prevent this from happening if you'd like.

When fall is in the air, nothing seems to hit the spot quite like pumpkin spice. These Pumpkin Spice Pancakes have just the right amount of spice to fill your kitchen with a great aroma when they're cooking. And if you think your kitchen smells good, wait until you taste them.

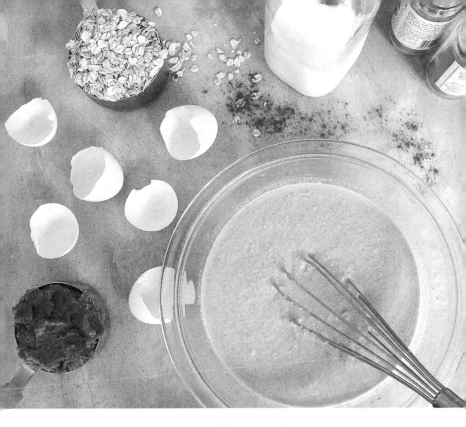

2. Blitz everything in the blender until you have a smooth liquid.
3. Pour the pancake mixture into a large bowl.
4. Let the batter rest for 5 to 10 minutes. This allows all of the ingredients to come together and gives the batter a better consistency.
5. Spray a non-stick skillet or griddle generously with vegetable oil and heat over medium heat.
6. Once the skillet is hot, add the batter using a ¼-cup measuring cup and pour the batter into the skillet to make the pancake. Use the measuring cup to help shape the pancake.
7. Cook until the sides appear set and bubbles form in the middle (about 2 to 3 minutes), then flip the pancake.
8. Once the pancake is cooked on that side, remove pancake from the heat and place on a plate.
9. Continue these steps with the rest of the batter.

Protein 8 grams | Carbs 33 grams | Calories 258

PUMPKIN SPICE PANCAKES

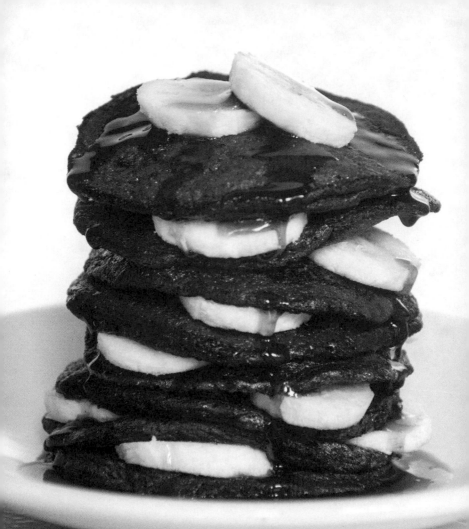

In the summer, a chocolate-covered frozen banana is the perfect treat. These Chocolate Banana Pancakes take that flavor combination to a different level. They're so easy to whip up and even easier to eat.

CHOCOLATE BANANA PANCAKES

MAKES 6 PANCAKES | SERVES 2

1 ripe banana, plus more to
   serve
2 large eggs
½ teaspoon baking powder

2 tablespoons unsweetened
   cocoa powder
Maple syrup, to serve

1. Add the banana to a bowl and mash it until it's nice and creamy—no lumps.
2. Crack the eggs into another bowl and whisk until they are thoroughly mixed.
3. Add the baking powder and cocoa powder to the bowl of banana and then pour in the eggs. Whisk to completely combine everything together.
4. Spray a non-stick skillet or griddle generously with vegetable oil and heat over medium heat.
5. Once the skillet is hot, add 2 tablespoons of batter into the pan to make the pancake.
6. Cook until the sides appear set (you won't see any bubbles), then carefully flip the pancake.
7. Once the pancake is cooked on that side, remove the pancake from the heat and place on a plate.
8. Continue these steps with the rest of the batter. Serve with sliced banana and maple syrup, if desired.

Note:
Because these pancakes are pretty thin, they scrunch up easily, and they're a little difficult to flip, I use a fork in addition to the spatula to help flip them over and remove them from the pan.

Protein 8 grams | Carbs 17 grams | Calories 135

VANILLA ALMOND PANCAKES

1 cup spelt flour
2 tablespoons sugar-free vanilla
  pudding mix
½ teaspoon baking powder
½ teaspoon baking soda
¾ cup plain Greek yogurt

½ cup + 2 tablespoons 2%
  low-fat milk
1 large egg
2 tablespoons maple syrup
¼ cup sliced almonds

---

1. Add the flour, pudding mix, baking powder, and baking soda to a bowl and whisk to combine.
2. In another bowl, whisk the yogurt, milk, egg, and maple syrup together until thoroughly combined.
3. Add the wet ingredients to the dry ingredients and whisk until thoroughly combined.
4. Stir in the almonds last.
5. Let the batter rest for 2 to 3 minutes. This allows all of the ingredients to come together and gives the batter a better consistency.
6. Spray a non-stick skillet or griddle generously with vegetable oil and heat over medium heat.
7. Once the skillet is hot, add the batter using a ¼-cup measuring cup and pour the batter into the skillet to make the pancake. Use the measuring cup to help shape the pancake.
8. Cook until the sides appear set and bubbles form in the middle (about 2 to 3 minutes), then flip the pancake.
9. Once the pancake is cooked on that side, remove pancake from the heat and place on a plate.
10. Continue these steps with the rest of the batter.

Protein 11 grams | Carbs 33 grams | Calories 238

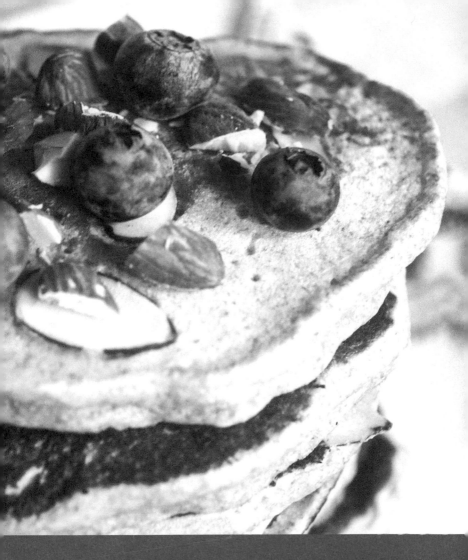

Vanilla and almond are subtle flavors that get added to recipes all the time, so why not pair the two flavors together? These Vanilla Almond Pancakes have the flavor of both with an added crunch from the sliced almonds. A great way to start the day. Serve with more sliced almonds and blueberries for extra flavor.

VANILLA ALMOND PANCAKES

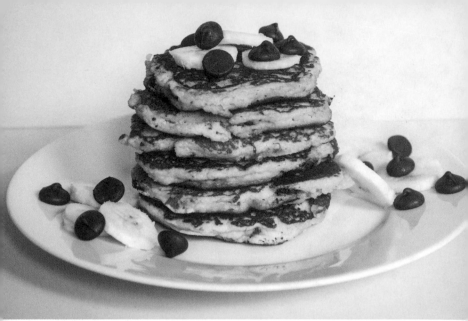

FUNKY MONKEY PANCAKES

1½ cups almond flour
1 teaspoon baking powder
1 teaspoon baking soda
¼ teaspoon salt
1 ripe medium banana, mashed,
    plus more to serve
2 large eggs, beaten

½ cup coconut milk
1 tablespoon maple syrup
1 teaspoon vanilla extract
½ cup chopped walnuts
½ cup dark chocolate chips,
    plus more to serve

1. Add the flour, baking powder, baking soda, and salt to a bowl and whisk to thoroughly combine.
2. In a separate bowl, whisk the mashed banana, eggs, coconut milk, maple syrup, and vanilla together.

3. Add the wet ingredients to the dry ingredients and whisk to thoroughly combine them.
4. Now whisk in the walnuts and chocolate chips and mix until everything is well blended.
5. Let the batter rest for 5 to 10 minutes. This allows all of the ingredients to come together and gives the batter a better consistency.
6. Spray a non-stick skillet or griddle generously with vegetable oil and heat over medium-high heat.
7. Once the skillet is hot, add the batter using a ¼-cup measuring cup and pour the batter into the skillet to make the pancake. Use the measuring cup to help shape the pancake.
8. Cook until the sides appear set and bubbles form in the middle (about 2 to 3 minutes), then flip the pancake. These pancakes can be a bit tricky to flip due to the batter being so wet and heavy.
9. Once the pancake is cooked on that side, remove pancake from the heat and place on a plate.
10. Continue these steps with the rest of the batter.
11. Serve with sliced bananas and chocolate chips.

Protein 14 grams | Carbs 30 grams | Calories 519

Just like your favorite ice cream, these pancakes are jam packed with banana, walnuts, and chocolate chips. These Funky Monkey Pancakes are a sweet treat for breakfast or even dessert.

VANILLA PANCAKES

1½ cups spelt flour
2 tablespoons sugar-free vanilla
   pudding mix
1½ teaspoons baking powder
1 teaspoon baking soda
½ teaspoon salt
2 large eggs, beaten

2 tablespoons coconut oil,
   melted
1 tablespoon vanilla extract
¼ cup maple syrup, plus more
   for serving
1¼ cups plain kefir

1. Add the spelt flour, pudding mix, baking powder, baking soda, and salt to a bowl and whisk to combine.
2. In another bowl, whisk the eggs, coconut oil, vanilla, maple syrup, and kefir together until they are well combined. The melted coconut oil might harden up when combined with colder ingredients, so you can slightly warm the kefir to help prevent this from happening if you'd like.
3. Add the wet ingredients to the dry ingredients and whisk until thoroughly combined.
4. Let the batter rest for 2 to 3 minutes. This allows all of the ingredients to come together and gives the batter a better consistency.
5. Spray a non-stick skillet or griddle generously with vegetable oil and heat over medium heat.
6. Once the skillet is hot, add the batter using a ¼-cup measuring cup and pour the batter into the skillet to make the pancake. Use the measuring cup to help shape the pancake.
7. Cook until the sides appear set and bubbles form in the middle (about 2 to 3 minutes), then flip the pancake.
8. Once the pancake is cooked on that side, remove pancake from the heat and place on a plate.
9. Continue these steps with the rest of the batter.

Protein 12 grams | Carbs 47 grams | Calories 347

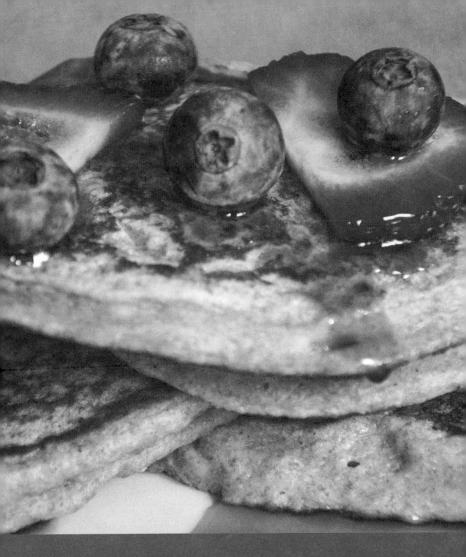

The subtle flavor of vanilla permeates these pancakes. They make for a perfect low-key morning breakfast, and topping them with maple syrup is the perfect way to serve them.

VANILLA PANCAKES

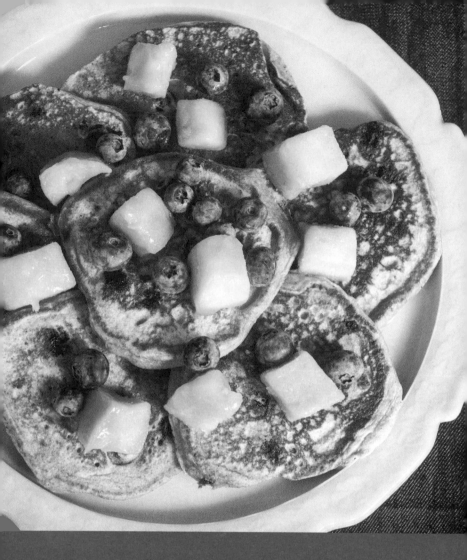

Did you ever think to combine blueberries with mangoes? Well you should, because they taste great together. The mango flavor in these pancakes is subtle, but it's there. Serve with fresh mango if you like. The blueberries add a great juicy pop of flavor to the light and fluffy pancakes.

BLUEBERRY MANGO PANCAKES

MAKES 8 PANCAKES | SERVES 4

1 cup spelt flour
½ teaspoon baking powder
½ teaspoon baking soda
¾ cup plain Greek yogurt
¼ cup + 2 tablespoons 2% low-fat milk

1 large egg
2 tablespoons maple syrup
½ cup puréed mangoes
½ cup blueberries

1. Add the flour, baking powder, and baking soda to a bowl and whisk to combine.
2. In another bowl, whisk the yogurt, milk, egg, maple syrup, and puréed mango together until combined.
3. Add the wet ingredients to the dry ingredients and whisk until thoroughly combined.
4. Carefully stir in the blueberries.
5. Let the batter rest for 2 to 3 minutes. This allows all of the ingredients to come together and gives the batter a better consistency.
6. Spray a non-stick skillet or griddle generously with vegetable oil and heat over medium heat.
7. Once the skillet is hot, add the batter using a ¼-cup measuring cup and pour the batter into the skillet to make the pancake. Use the measuring cup to help shape the pancake.
8. Cook until the sides appear set and bubbles form in the middle (about 2 to 3 minutes), then flip the pancake.
9. Once the pancake is cooked on that side, remove pancake from the heat and place on a plate.
10. Continue these steps with the rest of the batter.

Protein 10 grams | Carbs 37 grams | Calories 221

MOCHA PANCAKES

1½ cups spelt flour
¼ cup unsweetened cocoa
3 teaspoons instant espresso
  powder
1½ teaspoons baking powder
1 teaspoon baking soda

½ teaspoon salt
2 tablespoons coconut oil,
  melted
1 teaspoon vanilla extract
2 large eggs, beaten
1¼ cups plain kefir

1. Add the spelt flour, cocoa, espresso powder, baking powder, baking soda, and salt to a bowl and whisk to combine.
2. In another bowl, whisk the coconut oil, vanilla, eggs, and kefir together until they are well combined. The melted coconut oil might harden up when combined with colder ingredients, so you can slightly warm the kefir to help prevent this from happening if you'd like.
3. Add the wet ingredients to the dry ingredients and whisk until thoroughly combined.
4. Let the batter rest for 2 to 3 minutes. This allows all of the ingredients to come together and gives the batter a better consistency.
5. Spray a non-stick skillet or griddle generously with vegetable oil and heat over medium heat.
6. Once the skillet is hot, add the batter using a ¼-cup measuring cup and pour the batter into the skillet to make the pancake. Use the measuring cup to help shape the pancake.
7. Cook until the sides appear set and bubbles form in the middle (about 2 to 3 minutes), then flip the pancake.
8. Once the pancake is cooked on that side, remove pancake from the heat and place on a plate.
9. Continue these steps with the rest of the batter.

Protein 13 grams | Carbs 39 grams | Calories 317

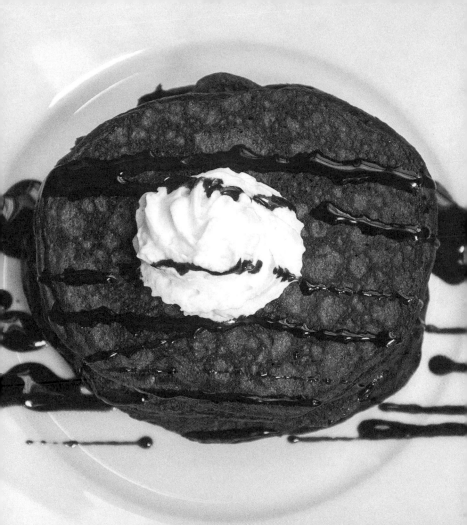

If you like coffee, and brunch is a regular word in your vocabulary, then these pancakes are for you. They're light and fluffy and full of coffee and cocoa flavor. Serve with a bit of whipped cream and chocolate syrup or shavings for the perfect topper.

MOCHA PANCAKES

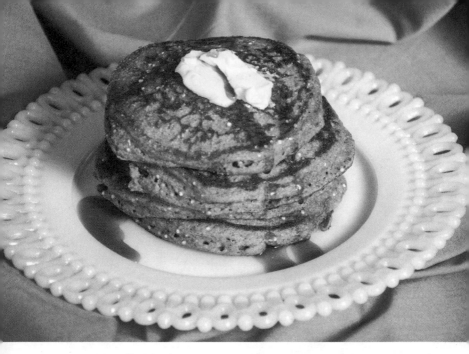

CHAI PANCAKES

MAKES 8 PANCAKES | SERVES 4

1½ cups quinoa flour
1½ teaspoons baking powder
1 teaspoon baking soda
1 teaspoon cinnamon
¾ teaspoon ground cardamom
Generous pinch ground cloves
½ teaspoon ground ginger
½ teaspoon ground allspice

½ teaspoon salt
2 large eggs, beaten
2 tablespoons coconut oil,
  melted
1¼ cups plain kefir
¼ cup maple syrup
1 teaspoon vanilla extract

1. In a large bowl, add the flour, baking powder, baking soda, cinnamon, cardamom, cloves, ginger, allspice, and salt together and whisk to thoroughly combine.
2. In another bowl, whisk the eggs, coconut oil, kefir, maple syrup, and vanilla together until combined. The

melted coconut oil might harden up when combined with colder ingredients, so you can slightly warm the kefir to help prevent this from happening if you'd like.

3. Add the wet ingredients to the dry ingredients and whisk until thoroughly combined.
4. Let the batter rest for 2 to 3 minutes. This allows all of the ingredients to come together and gives the batter a better consistency.
5. Spray a non-stick skillet or griddle generously with vegetable oil and heat over medium heat.
6. Once the skillet is hot, add the batter using a ¼-cup measuring cup and pour the batter into the skillet to make the pancake. Use the measuring cup to help shape the pancake.
7. Cook until the sides appear set and bubbles form in the middle (about 2 to 3 minutes), then flip the pancake.
8. Once the pancake is cooked on that side, remove pancake from the heat and place on a plate.
9. Continue these steps with the rest of the batter.

Protein 12 grams | Carbs 41 grams | Calories 332

These pancakes have the same spices as your favorite cup of chai tea. While you're cooking them, your kitchen will be filled with its warm fragrance. The flavor of these pancakes is subtle and the quinoa flour gives a slight crunch to the fluffy pancakes. These are best topped off with a pat of butter and maple syrup.

CHAI PANCAKES

CARROT CAKE PANCAKES

1½ cups old-fashioned rolled oats
1½ teaspoons baking powder
1 teaspoon baking soda
½ teaspoon cinnamon
¼ teaspoon salt
Dash of nutmeg
1 large egg

2 tablespoons coconut oil, melted
1 tablespoon maple syrup
1 teaspoon vanilla extract
1¼ cups 2% low-fat milk
1½ cups finely grated carrots
½ cup chopped golden raisins
½ cup chopped walnuts

1. Add all of the ingredients, except for the carrots, raisins, and walnuts, to a blender. The melted coconut oil might harden up when combined with colder ingredients, so you can slightly warm the milk to help prevent this from happening if you'd like.
2. Blitz everything in the blender until you have a smooth liquid.
3. Pour the pancake mixture into a large bowl.
4. Add the carrots, raisins, and walnuts to the batter and stir to thoroughly combine.
5. Let the batter rest for 5 to 10 minutes. This allows all of the ingredients to come together and gives the batter a better consistency.
6. Spray a non-stick skillet or griddle generously with vegetable oil and heat over medium heat.
7. Once the skillet is hot, add the batter using a ¼-cup measuring cup and pour the batter into the skillet to make the pancake. Use the measuring cup to help shape the pancake.

8. Cook until the sides appear set and bubbles form in the middle (about 2 to 3 minutes), then flip the pancake.
9. Once the pancake is cooked on that side, remove pancake from the heat and place on a plate.
10. Continue these steps with the rest of the batter.

Note:
Because of the extra moisture the carrots add to the batter, it may take a minute longer to cook on each side than other pancakes do.

Protein 11 grams | Carbs 50 grams | Calories 387

If you like carrot cake, you're going to love these pancakes. They're moist and rich with all of those flavors you love in carrot cake. While these look a little different than your traditional pancake (all of the bits of carrot show through the batter in these), the flavor will have you looking to slather these with cream cheese frosting. It's like cake for breakfast!

CARROT CAKE PANCAKES

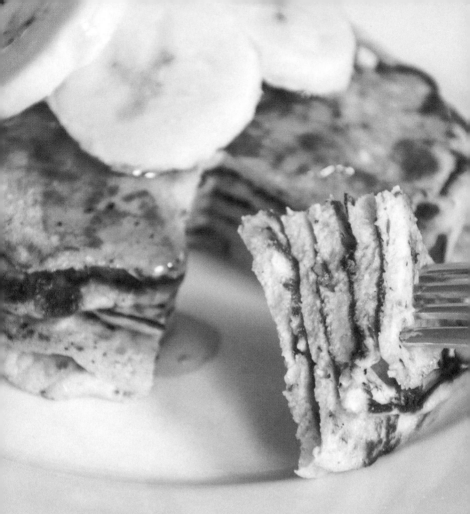

I thought that the basic 3-Ingredient Pancakes (page 30) needed a bit of a flavor boost. Mixing in a bit of honey made the pancakes sweeter, of course, but it added a little body too. The combination is fantastic and helps to up the overall taste of the basic 3-Ingredient Pancake. You can't go wrong serving these with sliced banana and honey.

HONEY BANANA PANCAKES

1 ripe banana, plus more for
  serving
2 large eggs

1 tablespoon honey
½ teaspoon baking powder
Maple syrup, for serving

1. Add the banana to a bowl and mash it until it's nice and creamy—no lumps.
2. Crack the eggs into another bowl and whisk until they are thoroughly mixed.
3. Add the honey and the baking powder to the bowl of banana and then pour in the eggs. Whisk to completely combine everything together.
4. Spray a non-stick skillet or griddle generously with vegetable oil and heat over medium heat.
5. Once the skillet is hot, add 2 tablespoons of batter into the skillet to make the pancake.
6. Cook until the sides appear set (you won't see any bubbles), then carefully flip the pancake.
7. Once the pancake is cooked on that side, remove the pancake from the heat and place on a plate.
8. Continue these steps with the rest of the batter.
9. Top with bananas and maple syrup.

Note:
Because these pancakes are pretty thin, they scrunch up easily, and they're a little difficult to flip. I used a fork in addition to the spatula to help flip them over and remove them from the pan.

Protein 7 grams | Carbs 22 grams | Calories 155

BANANA BLUEBERRY PANCAKES

1 cup spelt flour
½ teaspoon baking powder
½ teaspoon baking soda
1 ripe medium banana, mashed
¾ cup plain Greek yogurt

¼ cup + 2 tablespoons 2%
  low-fat milk
1 large egg
2 tablespoons maple syrup
½ cup blueberries

1. Add the flour, baking powder, and baking soda to a bowl and whisk to combine.
2. In another bowl, whisk the mashed banana, yogurt, milk, egg, and maple syrup until combined.
3. Add the wet ingredients to the dry ingredients and whisk until thoroughly combined.
4. Carefully stir in the blueberries.
5. Let the batter rest for 2 to 3 minutes. This allows all of the ingredients to come together and gives the batter a better consistency.
6. Spray a non-stick skillet or griddle generously with vegetable oil and heat over medium heat.
7. Once the skillet is hot, add the batter using a ¼-cup measuring cup and pour the batter into the skillet to make the pancake. Use the measuring cup to help shape the pancake.
8. Cook until the sides appear set and bubbles form in the middle (about 2 to 3 minutes), then flip the pancake.
9. Once the pancake is cooked on that side, remove pancake from the heat and place on a plate.
10. Continue these steps with the rest of the batter.

Protein 10 grams | Carbs 41 grams | Calories 234

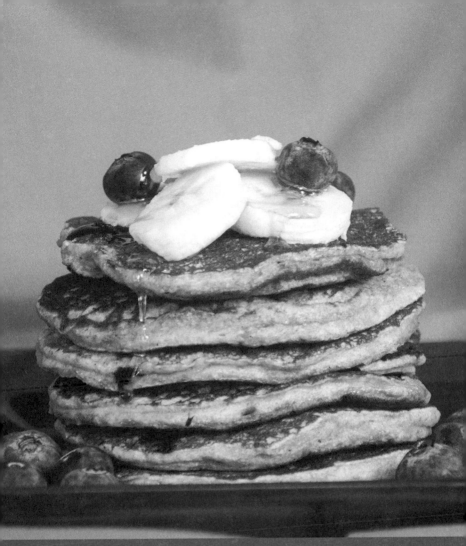

These light and fluffy Banana Blueberry Pancakes will keep you running all morning. Of course they're packed with protein, but they're also packed with flavor. Blueberries, bananas, and a drizzle of maple syrup are perfect toppings for these pancakes.

APPLE CINNAMON PANCAKES

1¾ cups old-fashioned rolled oats
1½ teaspoons baking powder
1 teaspoon baking soda
¼ teaspoon cinnamon
¼ teaspoon salt
1 cup applesauce

2 tablespoons coconut oil, melted
1 tablespoon maple syrup
1 large egg
1 teaspoon vanilla extract
½ cup 2% low-fat milk

1. Add all of the ingredients to blender. The melted coconut oil might harden up when combined with colder ingredients, so you can slightly warm the milk to help prevent this from happening if you'd like.
2. Blitz everything in the blender until you have a smooth liquid.
3. Pour the pancake batter into a large bowl.
4. Let the batter rest for 5 to 10 minutes. This allows all of the ingredients to come together and gives the batter a better consistency.
5. Spray a non-stick skillet or griddle generously with vegetable oil and heat over medium heat.
6. Once the skillet is hot, add the batter using a ¼-cup measuring cup and pour the batter into the skillet to make the pancake. Use the measuring cup to help shape the pancake.
7. Cook until the sides appear set and bubbles form in the middle (about 2 to 3 minutes), then flip the pancake.
8. Once the pancake is cooked on that side, remove pancake from the heat and place on a plate.
9. Continue these steps with the rest of the batter.

Protein 7 grams | Carbs 40 grams | Calories 280

Apples and cinnamon have been going along together forever. This flavor combination is perfect for breakfast, with a rich apple flavor and just a hint of cinnamon.

STRAWBERRY CHEESECAKE PANCAKES

MAKES 8 PANCAKES | SERVES 4

1 cup spelt flour
2 tablespoons sugar-free vanilla
   pudding mix
½ teaspoon baking powder
½ teaspoon baking soda
¾ cup plain Greek yogurt

½ cup + 2 tablespoons 2%
   low-fat milk
1 large egg
2 tablespoons maple syrup
1 cup thinly sliced strawberries

1. Add the flour, pudding mix, baking powder, and baking soda to a bowl and whisk to combine.
2. In another bowl, whisk the yogurt, milk, egg, and maple syrup until combined.
3. Add the wet ingredients to the dry ingredients and whisk until thoroughly combined.
4. Carefully stir in the strawberries.
5. Let the batter rest for 2 to 3 minutes. This allows all of the ingredients to come together and gives the batter a better consistency.
6. Spray a non-stick skillet or griddle generously with vegetable oil and heat over medium heat.
7. Once the skillet is hot, add the batter using a ¼-cup measuring cup and pour the batter into the skillet to make the pancake. Use the measuring cup to help shape the pancake.
8. Cook until the sides appear set and bubbles form in the middle (about 2 to 3 minutes), then flip the pancake.

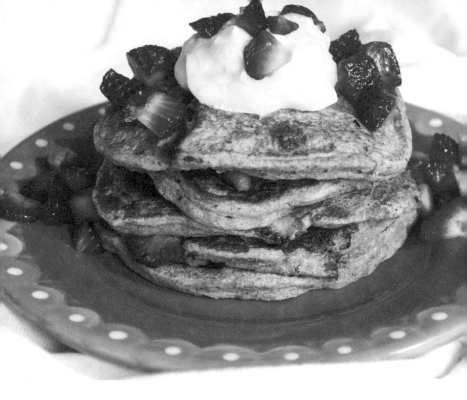

9. Once the pancake is cooked on that side, remove pancake from the heat and place on a plate.
10. Continue these steps with the rest of the batter.

Protein 10 grams | Carbs 34 grams | Calories 211

New York-style strawberry cheesecake is a classic dish. These Strawberry Cheesecake Pancakes give you a bit of that flavor without all the damage to your waistline. If you like, dress them up with some whipped cream and even more strawberries. Start your day with a smile with these lightly sweet pancakes.

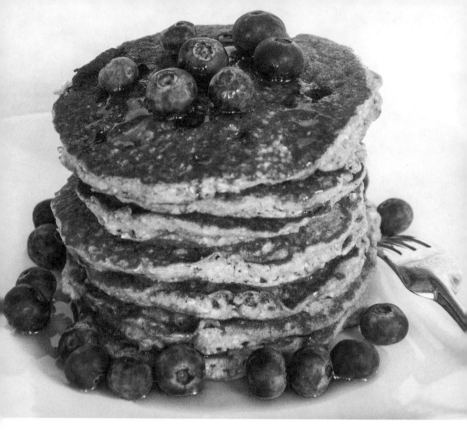

BLUEBERRY PANCAKES

MAKES 8 PANCAKES | SERVES 4

1¾ cups old-fashioned rolled oats
1½ teaspoons baking powder
1 teaspoon baking soda
½ teaspoon cinnamon
¼ teaspoon salt
1 large egg

2 tablespoons coconut oil, melted
1 tablespoon maple syrup
1 teaspoon vanilla extract
1¼ cups 2% low-fat milk
½ cup blueberries

1. Add all of the ingredients, except for the blueberries, to the blender. The melted coconut oil might harden up when combined with colder ingredients, so you can slightly warm the milk to help prevent this from happening if you'd like.
2. Blitz everything in the blender until you have a smooth liquid.
3. Pour the pancake mixture into a large bowl.
4. Carefully stir in the blueberries.
5. Let the batter rest for 5 to 10 minutes. This allows all of the ingredients to come together and gives the batter a better consistency.
6. Spray a non-stick skillet or griddle generously with vegetable oil and heat over medium heat.
7. Once the skillet is hot, add the batter using a ¼-cup measuring cup and pour the batter into the skillet to make the pancake. Use the measuring cup to help shape the pancake.
8. Cook until the sides appear set and bubbles form in the middle (about 2 to 3 minutes), then flip the pancake.
9. Once the pancake is cooked on that side, remove pancake from the heat and place on a plate.
10. Continue these steps with the rest of the batter.

Protein 9 grams | Carbs 34 grams | Calories 272

Sometimes there's nothing better than a simple blueberry pancake. Nothing fancy— just a light and fluffy pancake with the burst of blueberry in every bite. These pancakes fit that description to a T. The other great thing about these Blueberry Pancakes is that they come together quickly, so you can start eating them sooner. Serve them with maple syrup and even more blueberries.

BLUEBERRY PANCAKES

STRAWBERRY BANANA PANCAKES

MAKES 8 PANCAKES | SERVES 4

1 cup spelt flour
½ teaspoon baking powder
½ teaspoon baking soda
¾ cup plain Greek yogurt
1 ripe medium banana, mashed

½ cup + 2 tablespoons 2%
   low-fat milk
1 large egg
2 tablespoons maple syrup
¾ cup sliced strawberries

1. Add the flour, baking powder, and baking soda to a bowl and whisk to combine.
2. In another bowl, whisk the yogurt, mashed banana, milk, egg, and maple syrup until combined.
3. Add the wet ingredients to the dry ingredients and whisk until thoroughly combined.
4. Carefully stir in the strawberries.
5. Let the batter rest for 2 to 3 minutes. This allows all of the ingredients to come together and gives the batter a better consistency.
6. Spray a non-stick skillet or griddle generously with vegetable oil and heat over medium heat.
7. Once the skillet is hot, add the batter using a ¼-cup measuring cup and pour the batter into the skillet to make the pancake. Use the measuring cup to help shape the pancake.
8. Cook until the sides appear set and bubbles form in the middle (about 2 to 3 minutes), then flip the pancake.
9. Once the pancake is cooked on that side, remove pancake from the heat and place on a plate.
10. Continue these steps with the rest of the batter.

Protein 11 grams | Carbs 41 grams | Calories 242

HIGH-PROTEIN PANCAKES

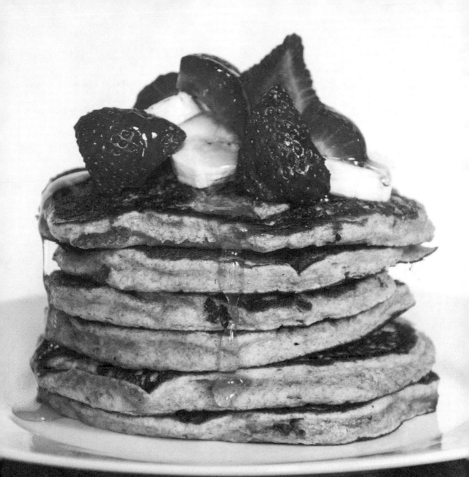

Strawberries and bananas are best friends. Those zingy strawberries paired with mellow bananas result in a flavor combination that's hard to beat. Throw in some protein-rich ingredients and you've got yourself a pancake that's healthy and delicious. Top these pancakes with maple syrup and more fruit.

PEACHES AND CREAM PANCAKES

1¾ cups old-fashioned rolled
  oats
2 tablespoons sugar-free vanilla
  pudding mix
1½ teaspoons baking powder
1 teaspoon baking soda
½ teaspoon cinnamon
¼ teaspoon salt

1 tablespoon butter, melted
1 large egg
¼ cup 2% low-fat milk
1 teaspoon vanilla extract
2 cups peeled and sliced
  peaches (if using frozen
  peaches, thaw them first)

1. Add all of the ingredients to a blender.
2. Blitz everything in the blender until you have a smooth liquid.
3. Pour the pancake batter into a large bowl.
4. Let the batter rest for 5 to 10 minutes. This allows all of the ingredients to come together and gives the batter a better consistency.
5. Spray a non-stick skillet or griddle generously with vegetable oil and heat over medium-low heat.
6. Once the skillet is hot, add the batter using a ¼-cup measuring cup and pour the batter into the skillet to make the pancake. Use the measuring cup to help shape the pancake.
7. Cook until the sides appear set and bubbles form in the middle (about 2 to 3 minutes), then flip the pancake.
8. Once the pancake is cooked on that side, remove pancake from the heat and place on a plate.
9. Continue these steps with the rest of the batter.

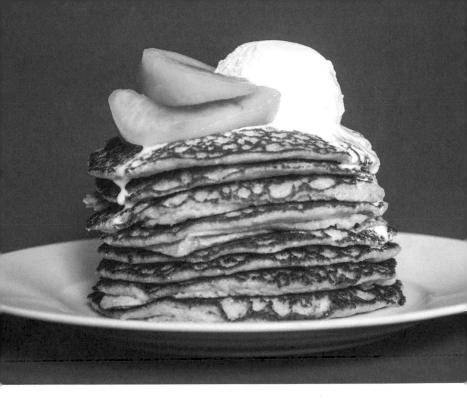

Note:

Because these pancakes have so much fruit in them, they take a bit longer to cook, so you'll want to cook them at a slightly lower temperature. That way you can cook them longer without burning the outer layer.

Protein 8 grams | Carbs 33 grams | Calories 215

Peaches and cream are an old-time favorite summer treat. These pancakes are filled with peaches and have a rich, creamy flavor from the vanilla pudding in the mix. They are best enjoyed when peaches are at their flavorful peak in the summertime. Fresh peaches and whipped cream are a perfect topping for these pancakes.

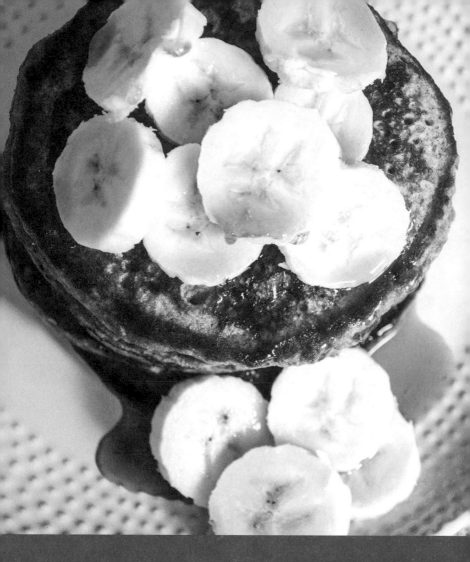

Banana bread makes a great-tasting snack, but why not have it for breakfast? These Banana Bread Pancakes will make you think you're eating that classic treat. Top with bananas and maple syrup.

HIGH-PROTEIN PANCAKES

BANANA BREAD PANCAKES

1 cup spelt flour
½ teaspoon baking powder
½ teaspoon baking soda
¾ cup plain Greek yogurt
1 ripe medium banana, mashed

½ cup + 2 tablespoons 2%
  low-fat milk
1 large egg
2 tablespoons maple syrup

1. Add the flour, baking powder, and baking soda to a bowl and whisk to combine.
2. In another bowl, whisk the yogurt, mashed banana, milk, egg, and maple syrup until combined.
3. Add the wet ingredients to the dry ingredients and whisk until combined.
4. Let the batter rest for 2 to 3 minutes. This allows all of the ingredients to come together and gives the batter a better consistency.
5. Spray a non-stick skillet or griddle generously with vegetable oil and heat over medium heat.
6. Once the skillet is hot, add the batter using a ¼-cup measuring cup and pour the batter into the skillet to make the pancake. Use the measuring cup to help shape the pancake.
7. Cook until the sides appear set and bubbles form in the middle (about 2 to 3 minutes), then flip the pancake.
8. Once the pancake is cooked on that side, remove pancake from the heat and place on a plate.
9. Continue these steps with the rest of the batter.

Protein 11 grams | Carbs 39 grams | Calories 231

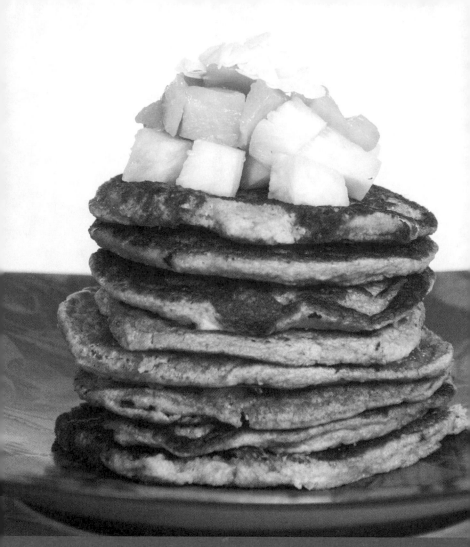

The next time you have breakfast, why not take a trip to the tropics? These Tropical Pancakes are full of coconut, banana, pineapple, and mango—and you can pile even more on top. These flavors combine to make you feel like you've left your kitchen and arrived on a lush island.

HIGH-PROTEIN PANCAKES

TROPICAL PANCAKES

1¾ cups old-fashioned rolled
  oats
1½ teaspoons baking powder
1 teaspoon baking soda
½ teaspoon cinnamon
¼ teaspoon salt
1 ripe medium banana, mashed
2 tablespoons coconut oil,
  melted
1 tablespoon maple syrup
1 large egg

1 teaspoon vanilla extract
¾ cup 2% low-fat milk
½ cup canned full-fat coconut
  milk
½ cup finely diced pineapple
  (if using frozen, make sure
  it's been thawed)
½ cup finely diced mango
  (if using frozen, make sure
  it's been thawed)

1. Add all of the ingredients, except the pineapple and mango, to a blender. The melted coconut oil might harden up when combined with colder ingredients, so you can slightly warm the milk to help prevent this from happening if you'd like.
2. Blitz the mixture in the blender until you have a smooth liquid.
3. Pour the pancake batter into a large bowl.
4. Stir in the pineapple and mango.
5. Let the batter rest for 5 to 10 minutes. This allows all of the ingredients to come together and gives the batter a better consistency.
6. Spray a non-stick skillet or griddle generously with vegetable oil and heat over medium-low heat.
7. Once the skillet is hot, add the batter using a ¼-cup measuring cup and pour the batter into the skillet to make the pancake. Use the measuring cup to help shape the pancake.

Continued

8. Cook until the sides appear set and bubbles form in the middle (about 2 to 3 minutes), then flip the pancake.
9. Once the pancake is cooked on that side, remove pancake from the heat and place on a plate.
10. Continue these steps with the rest of the batter.

Note:
Because these pancakes have so much fruit in them, they take a bit longer to cook, so you'll want to cook them at a slightly lower temperature. That way you can cook them longer without burning the outer layer.

Protein 9 grams | Carbs 44 grams | Calories 363

***Boldface** numbers indicate illustrations.